1—
18

The
7-Day
BACK PAIN
Cure

*How Thousands of People Got Relief
Without Doctors, Drugs, or Surgery...
and How You Can, Too!*

Jesse Cannone

How Thousands of People Got Relief Without Doctors, Drugs, or Surgery... and How You Can, Too!

Get more back pain tips, stretches, videos
and additional help online at:
www.losethebackpain.com/7DayCureSupport

JESSE CANNONE

Healthy Back Institute®

Austin

Copyright © 2009, 2011, 2015 Jesse Cannone
All Rights Reserved
ISBN Print
978-1-937445-11-9
ISBN Kindle/EBook
978-1-937445-12-6
Library of Congress Control Number: 2011937822

Published by The Healthy Back Institute®
141 E. Mercer Street, Suite E
Dripping Springs, TX 78620 USA
800-216-4908

Printed in the United States of America

WHAT OTHERS ARE SAYING ABOUT THE 7-DAY BACK PAIN CURE

Hi, I am a complementary Therapist here in the UK, and I make an effort to keep myself healthy, mind body and soul. Imagine the shock of suddenly losing my ability to stand and in excruciating pain, hit the floor for no reason at all. I couldn't move without screaming out. I went into shock; trembling and freezing cold. I just had no answers so, very reluctantly, called the doctor who didn't know anything about me. On his examination he said that I needed to take 2 sorts of his painkillers. Then if my pain didn't get any better, then he had something stronger and if that didn't work, IT WAS SURGERY!!! Fortunately I could still raise my head for a few minutes at a time, so I began to look through the internet search engine - sudden back pain - and I thank Yahweh for leading me to you. At first I thought you might be wrong, but sure enough, just following your advice with tiny exercises first, then progressing, the improvement was daily. I am now recommending you to everyone I contact.
- Loren Brown, Norwich, Norfolk, UK

I have had back pain for the last 15 years or so on a 24/7 basis. Needless to say, I have tried many means for some relief. I found this book written in everyday language and to be extremely informative. Written in an organized fashion, covering all causes of back problems and what could help the situation. It gave me a mental check list to see if I have covered all I can do. When you are in pain everything in life goes out the window. Depression sets in when you feel there isn't anything left to do. This book educates you and empowers you to find a means to get rid of that back pain.
- Annie

It is still early days for this plan with me. The physio has given me good exercises towards strengthening my muscles and encouraging me to listen to my body, but to persist. I had the cortisone epidural for pain with a herniated disc many years ago, and the doctor now says that the damage from that is now my worst problem with my back. There are other problems,

such as osteoarthritis. The pain has mostly gone. I am no longer so stiff when I stand for a time. I have pulled some weeds in the garden today, and do not feel the way I would have a month ago. Heal-n-Soothe tablets are doing more good than the Dr's prescription did, Rub On Relief at night lets me sleep better than for a long time. I intend to keep on with this program!
- Rosemary Martin "remanildra" (Melbourne Australia)

Two years ago I had major surgery regarding stenosis. A lot of pain, weakness, walking bent over associated with it. Was surprised to find a chapter in your book on stenosis. Have followed your recommendations and after two weeks I feel much improved! It may be beginners luck, too early to say but, in any event, I will continue with the exercises, Heal-n-Soothe, vitamins, and inversion. How good it feels to feel good. Two of my friends now have your book too. Thanks for your help.
- Gary G.

I was so relieved to read this book to find that there are alternative ways to help chronic back pain. I have had back problems since 1986, and have taken many different pain pills, therapy, and so many epidurals that are not effective for long time comfort. I have just ordered a week ago an Inversion Table, and after mentioning this to two orthopedic doctors they thought it was a good choice. If I get relieve from doing it, then I feel I am doing my body a great service by eliminating drugs, and steroids. Thank God there are people that look into, and research alternative methods. Having a positive attitude is also helpful for your nerve system.
- Irene

I have suffered with back pain since an auto accident in 1969. Nothing I have tried except for drugs has eased the pain. I do not like taking drugs so the strongest I take is Ibuprofen, and that I try to keep down to a minimum. Once I got connected with Jesse's programs I have been able to deal with my pain without any drugs, and having days without pain; especially using the inversion table! Thank you for all the information and products that have been sent my way.
- sugarmt

I have been in pain on and off for over 8 years now by using firstly, the digestive enzymes, choosing a chiro who understood about trigger point therapy and in conjunction with the Lose the Back Pain System, I have found a 80% reduction in pain and increased mobility. Direct no nonsense approach worked for me - well done guys!
- Frank Paul Strever, Perth, Australia

I purchased one bottle of your supplement about three weeks ago & I have to say I'm so impressed with the results that I could possibly be a sales rep for the product. You see, without going in a lot of detail, I've been in severe pain for about four yrs straight. I've done rounds of physical therapy, chiropractic, acupuncture, medicines, supplements, u name it but nothing has worked. Anyway, I've got to order more because I'm out but I even told my father about it who has RA & my granny & stepdad about it & want to provide them some pain relief. I want my life back! So I just want to thank you for your product & for first time HOPE of a better life.
- Crystal Evens

I really love this stuff! It has truly cured a year and a half worth of problems! WOW! By the way I'm an upcoming pro fighter, and I'm from the great Big state of TEXAS.
- Josh Tabor (Fighter), Haltom City, TX

This book is for YOU—the back pain sufferer who is tired of letting pain control your life. In these pages, you will find the keys to lasting relief.

CONTENTS

PART III:
PAIN RELIEF ACTION PLANS

PREFACE

Every back pain sufferer has a story. I'm no exception. Mine involves an attractive woman, a marathon, a surgeon, a chiropractor, and a remarkable and entirely unexpected solution to back pain that I popularized called Muscle Balance Therapy™.

As publisher of the Less Pain, More Life e-mail newsletter (www.losethebackpain.com), I'm often asked by many of my 600,000 readers worldwide how I became one of the leading experts on using nonmedical approaches to resolving stubborn, recurring back pain.

Here's what is, I hope, my interesting, but somewhat embarrassing, story.

Several years ago, I met a very attractive woman at the gym where I worked as a personal trainer. As every guy can tell you, sometimes we do stupid things to impress a girl, especially the woman of our dreams. For me, this was one of those times.

I asked Maria out on a date and held my breath, awaiting her answer. Much to my relief, she smiled and said she was interested.

Yes!

I gave myself mental high fives while pretending, of course, to be a cool customer. Maria asked if I wanted to go running with her.

Running? Oh, yeah, definitely. I love to run.

But Maria wasn't just any runner. Maria enjoyed marathons, all 26-plus miles of them. She wondered if I wanted to join her on one of her training workouts.

I smiled and agreed. Maria smiled back and then left. It was official. We had a date.

I felt terrific, except for one small problem. I wasn't actually a runner. But I couldn't admit that to Maria. I had my fragile male ego to consider! True, I was a personal trainer and a bodybuilder, but I was more into lifting weights than running. I'd never really run more than a mile or two. Still, I figured I could keep up—or rather, I was going to make darn sure I could.

Thankfully, my first run with Maria was great. We hit it off, and I handled the four-mile jaunt without a problem. Since I kept up so well, we scheduled another run—this time, for eight miles. Our budding romance bloomed, and my running shoes got a nice workout.

Then came our third run. Since I'd managed eight miles, Maria decided to take me for twelve. It wasn't easy, but I did finish. After all, my fragile male ego had to finish, right? Tongue hanging out, I succeeded and thought everything would be fine.

Maria and I then went to the local grocery store. We were having a great conversation when suddenly my left knee buckled and I fell to the floor. When I tried to get up, I fell back down again. How embarrassing. Here I was, a 22-year-old bodybuilder, lying on the ground in pain, unable to walk, and failing miserably to impress this attractive woman.

Several weeks went by, but my knee didn't get any better. Assuming I'd injured it, I visited multiple doctors, chiropractors, and orthopedic surgeons. My X-rays showed healthy bones. My MRI showed normal soft tissues. What was going on?

Even after multiple cortisone shots and tons of painkillers, the pain was still there. The orthopedic surgeon suggested surgery to "clean up" some of the debris in the fluid of the joint—even though other people with similar levels of debris experienced no pain.

I'd tried everything and still couldn't walk. Desperate, I scheduled the surgery.

Meanwhile, as part of an effort to expand my skills as a personal trainer, I was attending a seminar on fitness rehabilitation—a topic that now was even more relevant to my life. One of the presenters was a knee expert. After his talk, I spoke with him about my situation.

He examined me, observing how I stood and how I walked. When he finished, he looked at me and said, "You don't have a knee problem at all."

What? Obviously, this comment surprised me. But since the surgery was only a few days away, I asked him to continue.

"The muscles on the left and right sides of your body are not in balance," he said. "One side is much tighter than the other, and it's shifting most of your body weight to the left. That's why your left knee is bothering you. It's carrying most of your weight."

Because of this imbalance, he explained, I wasn't really walking with both legs, but actually just sort of hopping on one.

Hmmm...this might explain a lot.

Of course, I'd never heard of such a thing as muscles being out of balance. But it was what he said next that changed my life.

"Here, let me show you a stretch you can use to even out the difference in muscle flexibility between the left and right sides of your body. Try it."

I did what he suggested and within a few minutes felt a little better. I did that same stretch a few times every day for the next few days. Much to my surprise, my pain was 80 percent gone within three days and 100 percent gone within seven days.

Needless to say, I canceled my surgery!

As if this wasn't surprising enough, within a short period of time, two more of my other physical problems fixed themselves—scoliosis and back pain.

When I was an elementary-school student, I had been given a physical a few days before school started. I was diagnosed with a mild case of scoliosis—a slightly abnormal curvature of the spine. Rather than running straight up and down, my spine had a bit of an "S" curve to it—with one part bowing slightly to the right and the other slightly to the left. Most likely, this contributed to the second problem I had later in life—back pain.

When I became a bodybuilder, I began to develop problems

with my mid-back—the part between my shoulder blades. It always bothered me, but I couldn't figure out how to get rid of it. But now an unusual thing happened. When I did the stretches to rebalance the muscles that were causing the pain in my knee, I unintentionally eliminated my back pain, too.

In hindsight, I realized I never really had a knee problem, a back problem, or scoliosis. What I had was a muscle imbalance problem. One side of my body was tighter and less flexible than the other. This uneven tension pulled my spinal column to one side, causing what appeared to be scoliosis. This same tension compressed some of the nerves in my spine and in my mid-back region, causing my back pain. It also shifted my hips to favor one side of my body so that most of my body weight was borne by my left leg, and of course, my left knee.

When I ran the 12 miles, which was pretty ambitious in itself, I didn't really run 12 miles so much as hop 12 miles on one leg. Of course, after my initial collapse, when I should have given my knee a chance to rest, my muscles were still out of balance. Without realizing it, I kept putting all my weight on the bad knee just by walking through my daily life. It's amazing my knee held up as long as it did!

To make matters worse, the imbalanced muscles that were pulling unevenly on my bad knee caused the joint to operate out of alignment. It's like a car that has one tire half-filled with air. The whole car starts dragging to one side and all the parts wear unevenly until some part of the car breaks.

By stretching and doing rebalancing exercises, I was able to restore the balance in my muscles and body frame, eliminate my pain quickly, and go on to live pain free. I became fascinated with how such a simple solution as stretching and doing muscle-balancing exercises could be so effective. Why weren't my many doctors aware of this approach?

I began telling my friends and family about what had happened to me. They wanted to know how they could stop their back pain like I had. Despite my desire to help them, I couldn't point to any doctors, physical therapists, clinics, chiropractors, books, videos, or audiotapes that talked about this commonsense explanation of what causes back pain and how to get rid of it.

The more I shared my story, the more people wanted to learn about the solution I'd found. I felt angry and frustrated that this information wasn't being taught in medical schools or offered as an option ahead of drugs, shots, surgery, and other therapies that didn't take this imbalanced-body phenomenon into account.

I considered the possibility of trying to teach this form of self-treatment myself. But I'm not a medical doctor, orthopedic surgeon, chiropractor, or physical therapist (though I was getting close, as my personal-training practice had started to lean toward clients with back pain and injuries).

Really, who was going to take me seriously?

So, I did nothing and waited for the medical and chiropractic communities to catch up. I waited and waited and waited. Years went by, but nothing changed. My friends, family, and colleagues continued to get well- intentioned—but often incorrect—advice from people in positions of authority.

Finally, unable to continue watching people suffer needlessly, I got fed up. I decided to forget my insecurities about not being a medical doctor and try to help as many other back pain sufferers as I could—by teaching a solution I call Muscle Balance Therapy.

Since then, the company I founded, the Healthy Back Institute®, has helped over 565,385 people in 123 countries free themselves from the shackles of back, neck and other pain. Every month, thousands more discover how to treat themselves through my video training, self-diagnosis, and self-treatment kit, my free Less Pain, More Life e-mail newsletter, and many other resources, all of which can be found at www.losethebackpain.com.

This book is my most recent effort to prevent back pain sufferers like you from going through often unnecessary surgeries, injections, and drugs.

In these pages, I'll show you how to determine the underlying—and almost always hidden—causes of your back pain. Then I'll show you how to use that knowledge to get rid of most, if not all, of your pain, typically within seven days.

Of course, this estimate is just an average. Your case may be different. I've had clients who solved back pain problems they'd suffered with for 15 years within two days (definitely a best-case scenario).

Others took two or three weeks to get rid of 70 percent of their pain—a great outcome for those who had suffered daily for decades. In some rarer cases, clients had to use not only Muscle Balance Therapy, but a number of other approaches to get good results. If your situation happens to require "the kitchen sink," you'll find it in this book.

And don't worry—what you'll discover in the following pages will pass your "commonsense" test with flying colors. As you read, you'll find yourself nodding along and telling yourself, "Yes, this makes sense." But let me warn you in advance: Your doctor, chiropractor, massage therapist, or physical therapist may not be familiar with these principles. We'll get into why that's the case in later chapters.

So that's my story of how I accidentally and reluctantly became a widely followed expert on using non-medical approaches to eliminate stubborn, recurring back pain, and how I came to develop and popularize Muscle Balance Therapy.

Oh, and in case you're wondering what happened to Maria and me: She felt terribly guilty for the pain I suffered because of all that running. It certainly wasn't her fault, but she still took care of me during the weeks that followed my grocery store collapse. In the end, I guess I needn't have worried about it, as we continued to date each other and ultimately got married. Today, we have eight children in our happy family.

But enough about me. Let's get started on getting rid of your back pain so you, too, can live a pain free life.

PART I:

THE HIDDEN CAUSES OF BACK PAIN

CHAPTER 1

THE SEVEN BACK PAIN MISTAKES

The secret of success is learning how to use pain and pleasure instead of having pain and pleasure use you. If you do that, you're in control of your life. If you don't, life controls you.
Tony Robbins

If you're reading this book, most likely you—or a loved one—is experiencing, or has experienced, back pain. Maybe you've tried some of the treatments out there but haven't found any lasting relief. At this point, you may be wondering why you haven't had greater success. Through my practice, I've found that the reasons back pain sufferers continue to suffer are usually because they make one or more of the following seven common mistakes.

Mistake #1:
Continuing a Treatment That Doesn't Work

I've talked to a number of back pain sufferers who have amazing stories of how long they tried a particular type of treatment before giving it up. Prior to enlisting our help, one of our clients actually went through 70 treatments with a chiropractor—and experienced no relief at all.

I know of several other clients who spent a lot of money on massage therapists and acupuncturists, only to get temporary relief that disappeared within a few days.

This doesn't make any sense. If you're using a back pain solution that doesn't work or hasn't worked permanently, it's worth trying a different approach. Some treatments work for some people, but if a treatment isn't working *for you*, that's what's important.

Here's a general rule to follow: If you see no improvement after going through a three-month period of treatment, consider making a change. It's not so much that you should have only X amount of treatments, but that you should notice steady progress in your pain relief. This relief should be of the long-lasting variety—not the kind that wears off in a few hours.

Mistake #2:
Failing to Solve the Problem the First Time

Many people experience back pain that lasts a few days and then subsides. When the pain disappears, rather than make an effort to identify and address the cause of it, they simply forget about it.

Here's an example: About 10 years ago, my mother had her first bout with back pain. She suffered back spasms for a few days, then the pain went away and she went on with her life. Two years later, it came back—much worse than before. It got so bad that she couldn't work. If she had taken that first round of pain more seriously, I doubt she would have had to go through the second one. Even if she did, it wouldn't have been nearly as bad and she'd have known exactly what to do to get rid of the pain again, but this time much more quickly.

I understand why this happens. Most people believe that when the pain goes away, the problem does, too. This is a common misconception that I hope will be corrected as you read this book.

The truth is, even though the pain may ease up for a while, if you haven't figured out what caused it in the first place, that cause is still there, lurking, waiting to flare up again. Of course, figuring out what causes back pain isn't always easy.

If you have a fall or some other sudden accident, it's not difficult to figure out why your back hurts. But in nearly all cases, the pain is caused by any number of things, things you may not have even thought about. You need to investigate what unhealthy conditions may be developing in your body and, more important, what's creating those conditions. I like to call these "hidden causes," and you'll discover them later in this book.

Mistake #3:
Thinking You're Too "Healthy" or "Fit" to Have Back Pain

You may eat right, exercise regularly, and enjoy good health, but that doesn't mean you can't experience back pain. Having been a personal trainer for many years, I've seen a lot of people in excellent shape who suddenly find themselves with lower back trouble. *The reality is that people who exercise frequently are just as likely—if not more so—to develop back pain.* Certain groups of athletes—including runners, cyclists, swimmers, dancers, gymnasts, and bodybuilders—are prime candidates for back problems.

Cyclists, for example, spend hours in a hunched position—a position that's not natural for the body to maintain over long periods of time. This causes a number of problems, as you'll discover shortly. In addition, the constant repetitive motion of peddling a bicycle overworks one set of muscles while underworking another. These imbalanced behaviors are very common in many people, and frequently they create conditions in the body that lead to back pain.

The same thing can happen to nonathletes. Even if you don't do any of the above-mentioned activities, your workout program can create problems if you're concentrating too heavily on certain areas of your body—making the pain worse—while neglecting others. Being fit doesn't necessarily mean that your body is well-balanced or devoid of other causes that could lead to back pain.

Mistake #4:
Treating Only the Symptoms

The majority of the treatments people receive— including cortisone shots, anti-inflammatory drugs, ultrasound, electrical stimulation, and the like—address only the symptoms of pain. You must understand that pain is merely a signal that something is wrong. *Even if you get rid of the pain, the problem is still going to be there.*

Here's an illustration: Suppose the oil light comes on in your car. You could put a piece of duct tape over the light, which would eliminate the aggravation, but it won't solve the problem. Your engine is still going to need attention. And unless you do something about it, it's only a matter of time before it will break down.

It's the same with pain. You're hurting because your body is suffering some sort of stress or strain. If you don't address it, you'll continue on with your "oil light" lit, so to speak, until something breaks down. Unfortunately, such a breakdown is usually very painful.

Mistake #5:
Not Understanding That Back Pain is a Process

Most of the time, back pain, neck pain, and sciatica take weeks, months, or even years to develop. Usually, you're not aware of a problem until something starts to hurt. But rarely is back pain the result of a one-time incident. Barring an injury like a car accident, back pain typically doesn't happen overnight. And even if a fall or an accident did trigger pain for you, the fact is that before the event you likely had several "hidden causes" placing unnecessary strain on your body.

Consider this example. Many of us sit for hours a day, especially if we're required to work at a computer or be in the driver's seat of a car or truck. The body wasn't made to sit that long. (That's why we're seeing so many cases of back pain now compared to several decades ago.)

Sitting puts extra pressure on the spine. It also shortens the muscles in the front of our hips and the backs of our legs while weakening others, like the ones in the rear end and the abdomen. To make matters worse, most of us adopt poor posture when we're sitting. The shoulders round, the head juts forward, and the back curves like a "C." When we stand up again, we feel that tightness in the backs of our legs and in our hips, and most of us retain that stooped posture even when in the upright position.

Imagine that the front end of your car is out of alignment, which causes the tires to wear unevenly. This also can happen to your muscles. Doing one thing over and over (such as sitting with bad posture) can throw your body out of its proper alignment, forcing it to adapt and work at strange angles. After a long period of operating this way, certain muscles, tendons, ligaments, and joints wear down, while others that are barely used become stiff and weak. The end result of this long process is often a condition like back pain, but it also can manifest itself as many other conditions, such as foot pain, knee pain, hip pain, shoulder problems, carpal tunnel syndrome, and dozens of others.

Unfortunately, X-rays, MRIs, and CAT scans don't reveal much of the uneven wear and tear we're talking about here, so many people are unaware of what has caused their pain. Even after undergoing treatment that may give them some relief, they have failed to address the underlying causes, likely setting them up to deal with this problem for a very long time.

Mistake #6:
Believing There are No More Options Left

After suffering back pain for a while and trying various treatments, you may begin to believe you've "tried it all" and exhausted all your options. Soon you tell yourself that surgery is the only option left or—even worse—that you'll just have to learn to live with the pain.

If you've experienced little success, you may understandably feel tired of trying. My "message of hope," so to speak, is that pain is not your problem. Determining what is *causing* the pain is the problem. When you can get to the underlying, often hidden, cause of your back pain, it becomes much easier to treat successfully.

Most practitioners try to get rid of back pain without ever really trying to figure out what's causing it. For example, two people can experience the exact same level and location of back pain, but for wildly different reasons.

Let's say you've tried physical therapy, but it didn't work for you. It's not that physical therapy doesn't work; the problem is that the therapist didn't have you doing the right combination of things to address the specific causes of your pain. Remember: Pain isn't the problem. It's just a *message* that you have a problem.

Forget about treatments that simply try to make the back pain message go away. Until you've attempted to figure out what's causing the pain, you haven't come close to exhausting your treatment options. In fact, I'm willing to bet that there are several treatments you likely have not tried (maybe never even heard of), and I'll tell you about these later in this book.

Mistake #7:
Failing to Take Control

Many back pain sufferers look to others to make them well. The problem with this is that no one cares more about your body and health than you do, and in the end, you have to take the steps necessary to allow and assist your body to heal.

A medical doctor looks at back pain as a muscular problem.

Prescribe the right drugs, he believes, and the problem goes away.

The surgeon sees it as a disc or vertebrae problem—a bulging disc is putting pressure on a nerve. She thinks that by cutting away the problem, it will go away.

The acupuncturist feels that back pain is related to poor circulation within the body. By using acupuncture treatments, he encourages better circulation and believes that it will stimulate the body's natural self-healing powers to kick in.

The chiropractor sees back pain as a misalignment of the spinal column. She thinks that by manipulating the spinal column into alignment, she will fix the problem.

These treatment approaches are all partially right.

The challenge with back pain is that the cause is different for each person—and often involves a combination of factors. Because no back pain practitioner is well-versed in all these areas—nor overly knowledgeable about matching conditions with treatments—there's no one better than you to consider the "big picture," or holistic aspect, of what's causing your pain.

This is why I found relief only when I took charge of my own care. I certainly called on others when appropriate, but I was personally responsible and determined to get rid of the problem once and for all.

I encourage you to adopt the same attitude. As you read the chapters that follow, you'll come to understand what's going on with your body and learn how to finally get the lasting relief you've been looking for.

Let's get started!

Find out more about these
"seven mistakes" and how to avoid them
at: **www.losethebackpain.com/7mistakes**

CHAPTER 2

PAIN IS ONLY A SYMPTOM

*Pain is temporary. It may last a minute, or an hour,
or a day, or a year, but eventually it will subside and something
else will take its place. If I quit, however, it lasts forever.*
Lance Armstrong

Pain. It's a powerful word that creates strong feelings. Think back to the last time you experienced pain. If you're like most people, you probably remember some event that caused it—a paper cut, a sprained ankle, or a skinned knee.

Most people believe that back pain operates the same way—that it's caused by some isolated event. They "throw out" their backs, for instance, experience pain, and then have a back pain problem. Since the pain happened rather suddenly, they imagine that if they can get rid of the pain, they'll get rid of the problem.

Like many things in life, the real story is more complicated. Back pain is just a symptom that can be caused by many different things.

Two people can feel the exact same type of back pain for two entirely different reasons. If they were both to undergo the same treatment, one may start to feel better, but the other may not. It all depends on why the pain exists in the first place.

Let's say you have a dog, and one night that dog comes in whining. You know he's in pain, but you don't know why. Pain is just a sign that something is wrong.

Next, you may notice he's limping, which is a good sign that the pain is probably in his leg somewhere, but you still don't know what's causing it. To find out, you need to do some investigating.

Most likely, you would call your veterinarian and work toward finding a solution. You would not, in most cases, give the dog a pain reliever or a massage and then forget about it. Even if your dog felt better the next day, it's likely you would still want to be sure his leg was all right. Unfortunately, you might not treat yourself with the same care.

Many traditional back pain treatments focus primarily—if not exclusively—on just getting rid of the pain.

In the process, they fail to identify the underlying cause of that pain. Of course, it's great to have pain erased or, at least, diminished. But easing the pain without solving the problem means one thing— the pain comes back. That's why a lot of people seem to frequently "throw out" their backs and experience persistent, recurring back pain.

Pain is a Message...So Listen!

Pain is your body's way of telling you that something is out of balance or "messed up" in some way. That may not be the technical term doctors use, but it's the most accurate one I can think of!

Through pain, your body is trying to send a message that something is wrong and it needs help. When the message is silenced but the underlying problem is ignored, the communication has failed. Consequently, your body starts to "yell" louder by giving you more pain—recurring and more severe pain.

Your body is trying to tell you something, but you aren't listening!

In a healthy state, the body is usually pain free. Sure, there are the occasional times when a slight injury causes our otherwise healthy bodies to hurt, but in that situation we know precisely why we hurt—that's not always true with back pain, though. When we feel pain or stiffness in the back, neck, or shoulders, we attribute it to something—*I slept wrong, I moved the couch and threw out my back*—even if those aren't the true reasons why we're feeling pain.

That's because it's human nature to want to know the reason why we're in pain. Even if we don't know the cause, that's no reason to shrug off the pain—eventually, it's going to demand that we acknowledge it.

Pain can be as small as a nuisance—an ache or a stiffness—or it can be debilitating and all consuming. It's there for one purpose, and that is to alert us that something is wrong with our body. Pain is a warning that is sent to the brain telling us that something is wrong so we can do something about it. This message is sent by nerves into the spinal cord, which carries it to the brain. When you take pain medication, you're not curing the problem that caused the pain. You're merely blocking the message from being transmitted to your brain or you're reducing the effect that it has on your body.

So, if you can reduce or eliminate any pain by popping a pain pill or aspirin, is that enough? No, it's not. Until you heed the warning the pain is sending to your brain and cure the problem, the pain will continue to come back...it's your body's way of protecting itself. In that sense, pain is a good thing! Without it, we wouldn't know that something is wrong. Without pain, we wouldn't know when we're ill or that we have a broken bone, a sprained ankle, or a head injury. We then wouldn't seek the treatment that we need to heal and return to our otherwise healthy state. By neglecting to heed the warning that pain sends to the brain, the injury or illness that caused the pain in the first place can become much more significant through misuse, overuse, or neglect.

So when your body tells you that it's in pain, listen. Pain isn't the problem—it's a natural, internal signal that's telling you there is a problem so you can do something to correct it.

CHAPTER 3

SIX BACK PAIN MYTHS

*We must not be hampered by yesterday's myths
in concentrating on today's needs.*
Harold S. Geneen

Six Big Myths About Back Pain

What I want to emphasize here is that we can't just focus on symptoms like pain. Instead, we must turn our efforts toward figuring out and fixing the underlying problem causing the pain. Before I explain the primary causes, however, let me start by dispelling a few popular myths.

Myth #1:
You "Throw Out" Your Back

In the course of my work, I've taught hundreds of thousands of people my back pain treatment approach. When I ask them what's wrong, they almost always say something like, "I was doing X when I 'threw out' my back."

Usually, some physical activity precedes the back pain, like picking up a heavy object, sneezing, bending over, or getting out of bed. The thinking goes, "Well, since I didn't have pain before the activity, the activity must have caused the pain."

As you'll see in the next few chapters, the reality is a bit more complicated. In many cases, a physical activity can trigger a pain episode, but by itself, it isn't the underlying cause.

Consider this example: Let's say you fill a room with natural gas and then toss a match inside. You could say that the match caused the explosion, but it would be more accurate to say the match "triggered" or ignited the explosion. The better question to focus on is "Where did all that gas come from in the first place?"

It's very similar with back pain. A physical activity can trigger a pain episode, but it's not the "fuel" behind it. If you don't get rid of the underlying problem, then any number of things can "trigger" the pain.

Myth #2:
Back Pain Means Something is Wrong with the Back

People usually think that if they have back pain, their bodies are suffering from some mechanical dysfunction. "Since my body hurts," they say, "it must mean something is wrong with my body—something with the bones, the muscles, or the soft tissue that connects them."

While this is sometimes, if not often, the case, it's not the only underlying cause of back pain. Other factors that originate in your mind (e.g., stress levels), as well as your diet (unhealthy foods), can cause severe back pain episodes, even when there's nothing wrong with your spine, discs, joints, muscles, or ligaments. These factors also can exacerbate physically caused back pain, making it many times more painful.

Myth #3:
Current Pain Isn't Related to Previous Bouts

If you experienced a back pain episode two months ago and another today, you're likely to think these episodes are unrelated. Perhaps the last time it happened because you sneezed. This time you were moving furniture.

For most people, the trigger that causes their pain episode is different on different occasions. Naturally, they associate the "cause" to the trigger and believe the episodes are unrelated.

In fact, in the vast majority of cases, multiple back pain episodes are caused by the same underlying problem—even if each pain episode had a different trigger.

Let's consider again the room filled with natural gas—a dangerous situation, no doubt. But the gas is the source of the danger, not the match, static cling, or a cell phone ring that might create a spark to trigger the explosion.

The same is true when it comes to back pain. Once you've created conditions in your body, inadvertently or otherwise, that are ripe for an explosive bout of back pain, any number of things can set off a pain episode. Different activities that may trigger pain are only sparks igniting the gas that was there all along.

Myth #4:
Being Overweight is a Major Cause of Back Pain

Being overweight can contribute to back pain, but in most instances, it's only a minor cause of it. That's because the spine and back muscles are designed to carry the body, small or large. Our muscles may have to work harder to carry and move around extra poundage, but as long as everything is in balance, that extra weight shouldn't be the major cause of any back pain.

While being overweight is usually not the reason a person has back pain, it can create an extra burden for those who do have back problems—making it a little more difficult to exercise and move around when pain strikes.

It's important to note that while maintaining a healthy weight is highly encouraged for improving overall body health, when it comes to back pain, it might be just as important to worry about what you eat. Stick to healthy foods (see Chapter 8) and drink plenty of water to remove toxins from your body and promote blood flow. A healthy diet can play a more significant impact on reducing back pain than losing a few pounds.

Note: I should mention that unbalanced weight can cause back problems and back pain. This is particularly true for pregnant women, who are known to suffer from lower back pain. The reason for that pain is not because the baby is pressing on the mother's back, as many believe. It's due to an imbalance. As the baby grows, its weight pulls the mother forward. In response, the mother-to-be throws her shoulders and upper body back in an attempt to create balance. This compensation puts pressure on the mother's pelvis and lower back, creating back pain.

Myth #5:
Inactive People are More Likely to Have Back Pain

Because active people are perceived to be stronger than inactive people, it's believed that they are less likely to have injuries or illnesses which would cause back pain. Surprisingly, that's not true at all. In fact, the opposite is true—people who are most active suffer from back pain more often than couch potatoes. Not only are they more likely to have back pain, but their back pain is more frequent and at higher levels than their inactive counterparts.

When we think of inactive people, we tend to envision weakness—weak muscles, endurance, etc. However, active people and athletes conjure a different image—one of strength and power. The misconception relating to back pain, though, is because most back pain isn't caused by weakness—it's caused by muscle imbalances, injuries, or illness.

Simply stated, active people put themselves in a greater likelihood to experience back pain because they strain and overexert their bodies more frequently. I'm proof—my back and knee pain occurred when I was very active, pushing myself to run greater lengths than ever before. Because the muscles on one side of my body were weaker than the other side, my body was out of balance...the more active I was, the worse it got, finally resulting in extreme and sudden pain.

Myth #6:

The Best Thing for Back Pain is Bed Rest

Severe back pain may constitute the need for limited mobility and bed rest, but in the long run, significant bed rest can actually cause more pain and problems. Faster healing occurs when you take measures to treat the cause. This includes exercise and activities to increase your blood flow, range of motion, and flexibility.

However, there are multiple stages of healing and the best treatment is often determined by what stage of pain and healing you're currently in. Rest can be helpful at the outset of an acute back pain flare-up. Corrective stretches and exercises may be intolerable at this point so you need to start where you are and address the acute inflammation and severe pain first.

During later stages of recovery—especially when you've experienced chronic pain for months or years—additional treatments will become more important as you progress through the treatment cycle. Bed rest, on the other hand, can be detrimental at this point.

Too much time spent in bed can prolong your pain and healing time. It can also cause muscles to weaken over time, resulting in an increased chance for further injury. So, some activity is encouraged, even if it's just getting out of bed and walking to a chair and sitting up for half an hour. It will help keep you mobile and limber, and it will make your recovery shorter and more tolerable.

CHAPTER 4

TWO TYPES OF PAIN

*The best and most efficient pharmacy is
within your own system.*
Robert C. Peale

There are Two Types of Pain:
Which are You Suffering From?

Though there are many back pain conditions, such as sciatica, scoliosis, and a herniated disc, we can narrow them down to two basic categories: nerve-based pain and tissue-based pain.

You may have one or the other, or you may have both. Some treatments will ease nerve pain, others improve tissue pain. Some might, in some cases, work for both. But determining the right treatment for your particular case can require some investigation. This is, incidentally, why so many back pain sufferers find inconsistent relief.

Let me explain the differences between the two types of pain.

As the name suggests, nerve-based back pain is caused by a nerve that's not happy for some reason. Typically, it's being pressured, pinched, compressed, or injured in some way—usually by a nearby muscle or bone.

For example, if a nerve is surrounded by or next to a muscle that's unusually tight and inflexible, that muscle presses on the nerve, causing it to hurt. This is common in sciatica.

If a nearby piece of bone, such as a vertebra in your spinal column, is out of position, it also might press on the nerve, causing pain. These bones themselves may be out of position due to an overly tight or inflexible muscle nearby. In other words, the whole process may start with a tight muscle but end with a nerve that's irritated by a bone.

Nerve pain often, but not always, is felt as a burning, tingling, sharp, shooting, electrical, or numb sensation, or like "pins and needles."

Tissue-based pain, on the other hand, originates in the muscles, tendons, ligaments, or other connective tissues in the body. (Most commonly, the pain originates in the muscles.) Think back to the last time you gave someone a neck or back massage. You may recall feeling one or more "knots" in the muscles. These knots are one of the main causes of tissue-based pain. One way to tell if a knot is really a knot, or just a bone, is to see if it exists on both sides of the body in the exact same position. If it appears on both sides, it might be a bone or part of a joint. If it only appears on one side, it's more likely a knot.

This knot is more formally known as a "trigger point." I don't know why it's called this, but I suspect it's because if you press firmly on it, it triggers pain. Trigger points also are known to trigger pain in areas of the body other than where they're located, and this is called "referred pain."

A trigger point is caused in part by a pooling of toxins in your muscle tissue—which, in turn, is usually caused by imbalances in your diet, excess negative stress, and/or damage to the actual muscle fibers as a result of an injury, excessive exercise or physical activity.

If you're under a lot of stress, for example, your body's natural tendency is to shift to more shallow breathing and to "freeze" parts of your upper body (clenched jaws and tense shoulders are a few examples). This "freezing" reduces the amount of oxygen in your body and slows the circulation of blood in certain areas—such as your back. Without the optimal level of oxygen from deep breathing and without natural body movement to keep the blood flowing, toxins get "stuck" within tight muscle tissue. If this is allowed to continue for a long enough period of time, a trigger point develops, causing pain.

Trigger points also might be caused by an imbalance in the diet. For instance, many people who have been led to believe they aren't getting enough calcium may, in fact, be deficient in magnesium. Without magnesium, the body can't process calcium as it should. Magnesium also is involved in the muscle-relaxation response, so if the body doesn't have enough of it, trigger points are more likely to develop. Since proper muscle function depends on both calcium and magnesium—and since they depend on each other for absorption into the body's cells—an adequate, balanced supply (along with potassium and other trace minerals) is necessary for healthy, pain free muscles. Studies have shown that supplementing with these nutrients can help ease trigger points.

Another way to really aggravate trigger points is to drink too little water. When you're dehydrated, your blood doesn't have enough fluid to flush out all the toxins and other biological waste that your body produces. Under normal conditions, the blood washes away all these waste products, moving them to the liver and kidneys, where they are eliminated from the body.

But if you're even slightly dehydrated, there isn't enough water in your blood to do a good cleaning job in the little spaces between the cells that make up your muscles. When this happens, you're much more likely to develop trigger points—or if you already have them, they increase in size, severity, and pain.

Other types of tissue-based pain, such as pulled or strained tendons or ligaments, also can be caused by overuse. While a sudden trauma or injury can pull a ligament—an extreme form of overuse—doing the same type of moderate-intensity activity too many times can strain a tendon or ligament, too. There is a fine line between using and over-using your tendons and ligaments.

Notice how similar types of sharp, shooting pain—a trigger point in the muscle, an inflamed tendon, or a compressed nerve—can be caused by entirely different reasons. As you'll see in the next chapter, this is quite common. You also will see that if you don't know what's causing your pain, you could easily choose the wrong treatment approach!

You may already have an idea which type of pain you have. If not, you'll figure it out as you go through this book. For now, just remember that you need to know what's causing the pain before you can reasonably expect to get rid of it.

Find out why you're still in pain and what
you can do about it in this video:
www.losethebackpain.com/stillinpain

The Three Causes of All Back Pain

As I mentioned earlier, most people think they "throw out" their backs and then experience back pain. While you now know that this isn't the case, let's look at what does cause back pain.

All back pain comes from one of three sources—and these are almost always overlooked by doctors and other health care professionals. We'll discuss this in depth in the next chapter.

CHAPTER 5

THE THREE HIDDEN CAUSES OF ALL BACK PAIN

The man who has sufficient power over himself to wait
until his nature has recovered its even balance is the truly wise man,
but such beings are seldom met with.
Giacomo Casanova

Let me introduce to you to the three hidden causes of all back pain (really all health conditions, for that matter). I'll begin with terms that are slightly technical, and then explain what they mean in plain English. Once you understand these key concepts, you'll probably never look at your own back pain the same way again.

All back pain is ultimately caused by one (or more) of the following three issues:

1. Excess ("too much")
2. Deficiency ("too little")
3. Stagnation ("too slow")

All these terms revolve around the idea that to live pain free, you need to maintain a delicate balance in your body, mind, and diet. It's important to avoid too much (i.e., excess) of anything that causes you pain or too little (i.e., deficiency) of something in order to prevent pain from occurring.

For example, if you do too much weightlifting, causing your

muscles to get shorter and less flexible, and you do too little stretching to lengthen and increase the flexibility of your muscles, you create a condition that is ripe for back pain.

Similarly, if you have too much negative emotional stress and too little downtime to process and deal with that stress, you'll create conditions in your body that are ripe for pain, while limiting your ability to heal.

Let's look at each of these three concepts in more detail.

Excess: Too Much of Something

When we talk about excess, we're talking about too much of something. If you drink too much soda, coffee, or caffeinated drinks, you'll have too much caffeine in your system (as well as other junk). Since caffeine is a diuretic that causes you to urinate a lot, you'll have too little water left in your body. The discs in the spine need water to stay healthy and function optimally. Too little water and they degenerate, bulge, or herniate, making you vulnerable to nerve compression and pain.

If you eat too much of the wrong kinds of fats—such as hydrogenated (partially or fully) vegetable oils; fried foods; and foods such as chips, crackers, and the like— you'll likely carry too much fat on your body, potentially straining your muscles and putting extra pressure on your back. In addition, since the body requires a delicate balance of different kinds of fats to avoid inflammation, too much of these "bad" fats will tip the scales in favor of inflammation and pain. (I'll explain more about diet and inflammation in a later chapter.)

We can have too much of just about anything in any area of our lives. I've touched on diet, but what about the physical body? Too much running, cycling, or weightlifting—without cross-training with other types of exercise, sports, or activities—can lead to uneven muscle strength and flexibility.

Too much sitting at the computer can lead to shortened muscles in the backs of the legs, which creates back pain. Too much stretching, without strength training, can lead to weak and flabby muscles that no longer support the body properly.

We can expand this concept to our mental lives. Too much stress can weaken the body's defenses and lead to sickness. Too much anxiety can lead to tension headaches and irritable bowels—even panic attacks. Too much self-judgment can lead to depression and low self-esteem, which decreases blood flow in the body and robs the tissues of adequate oxygen supply.

All these excesses throw the body and mind out of balance, tipping the scales toward back pain—not to mention other kinds of pain and disease.

Deficiency: Too Little of Something

When we talk about deficiency, we're talking about too little of something. If you drink too little water, you run the risk of dehydration and toxic buildup in the body, as well as constipation and back pain. Eat too little fruits and vegetables, and your body doesn't get enough of the vitamins and minerals it needs to stay healthy, fight off stress, and lower your risk of experiencing back pain.

As with "too much," we can have "too little" of just about anything in any area of our lives. If we consider the physical body, the first deficiency that comes to mind is too little exercise. In America, we're suffering from an obesity epidemic. I talked about too much of the same kind of exercise a moment ago, but for many people, the problem is too little exercise. We're moving around a lot less than we used to and performing far fewer manual tasks, which is creating all kinds of aches and pains, to say nothing of the increase in such weight-related disorders as diabetes and heart disease.

If we consider our emotional lives, we can see how an insufficient amount of quiet time is a problem for many of us. We're bombarded by stimulation from all corners of our existence—televisions, cell phones, traffic noises, loud voices, radios, stereos, text messages, e-mails, and more. Rarely do we take the time to go to a quiet place and reflect.

This constant stimulation leaves us anxious and unable to relax, reducing the amount of oxygen that reaches the muscles and creating blood circulation that's too slow.

These deficiencies create an imbalance in the mind, body, and diet—again, setting us up to suffer because of some upcoming disorder or pain condition.

Stagnation: Something is Moving Too Slow

Stagnation can be caused by too much or too little of something in your life—or by both. Simply put, it's the slowdown of blood flow and body energy.

In a healthy body, the blood flows freely throughout the veins and arteries, supplying all organs and tissues with the oxygen and nutrients they need, while carrying waste away. However, if that blood flow is restricted somehow, say, in a trigger point within one of your back muscles, it slows down and clogs up the system.

Imagine one side of a two-lane highway. As long as those two lanes stay open, traffic flows freely (usually!). However, during times of construction, one lane often is closed, which narrows the passage-way and forces all the cars into the remaining lane. The flow slows down.

There are many causes of stagnation. Too much anxiety, tension, and fear all restrict blood vessels, as evidenced by the feeling of "cold hands." Too much sitting for long periods of time, whether at the computer or on an airplane, restricts the blood flow in your legs, and can even result in a clot. Too much "bad fat" in the diet can slow down blood flow and leave you fatigued. Too much strain on a muscle can cause a muscle spasm, which can restrict blood flow. Too little activity, too little stress relief, too little water, and too little stretching to elongate the muscle fibers all can lead to low energy and poor circulation. And poor circulation can lead to muscle soreness, toxin buildup, and back pain.

A Dangerous Cycle

It's easy to understand how these three points—too much, too little, and too slow—can all interact and feed each other. You can see how too much of one thing often prompts too little of something else—with the entire chain of too much and too little resulting in energy and blood flow that is too slow, creating back pain.

Suddenly it becomes clear why the more common approaches to treating back pain—those that focus strictly on pain—don't address the underlying conditions.

It's a dangerous and self-reinforcing cycle. Reversing excesses, deficiencies and stagnations to break the cycle of pain takes time and focused effort—but pays off with a healthier, more vibrant life as you recover.

Find out why you're still in pain and what
you can do about it in this 3-part video series:
www.losethebackpain.com/causesvideo

How to Get Out of the Pain Cycle

To understand how to get out of this cycle, let's look in more detail at the three key areas of your life that are impacted by the "too much/too little/too slow" causes of back pain. These are body, mind, and diet.

CHAPTER 6

THE BODY: THE PHYSICAL CAUSES OF PAIN

Illness is the most heeded of doctors: to goodness and
wisdom we only make promises; pain we obey.
Marcel Proust

In the previous chapter, we talked about how the causes of back pain are "too much" (excess) of something, "too little" (deficiency) of something, or blood circulation that's "too slow" (stagnation). Also, it's important to remember that you often will find a combination of several causes that are all working together to keep you in pain.

In this chapter, we'll focus on how these key concepts are related to your physical body. For most people, it all starts the same way. You use your body in an unbalanced manner, likely without being aware of it. For example, you may sit in a chair or car seat 10 hours a day, but stand or walk only an hour or two.

Next, one of two things happens. Some people develop tissue-based pain, which originates in the muscles, tendons, ligaments, or joints. Others suffer from nerve-based pain, a result of taut muscles pressuring a nerve or pulling the body out of alignment so the bones in the spinal column (or a joint) compress or pinch a nerve or force a disc to bulge or herniate. Often, people suffer from both types of pain at the same time.

Let's examine how these situations can develop.

Muscle Imbalances:
The Tug of War Inside Your Body

Human beings are born with well-balanced bodies, but rarely do they stay that way. Throughout our lives, we learn to use our muscles to master various activities, but because we tend to favor one side, or do some activities over and over again, we work some muscles too much and others too little.

Take our modern-day sedentary lifestyles, for example. Most of us sit far more than we stand or engage in activity. We sit at the computer, in a plane, in meetings, while watching TV, and while eating, driving, and visiting. If we were to log the hours we spend sitting, as opposed to other activities, we'd probably find that sitting takes up the majority of our time. We're a society of "too much" sitting— especially compared to 50 or 100 years ago.

Sitting, however, isn't the only way we use our muscles too little or too much. Consider the course of your own typical day. Most likely you use one hand more than the other to brush your teeth, style your hair, write, and eat. That hand and arm also are probably more prominent in activities such as cleaning, cooking, and doing laundry. When you drive, you use the right leg for both pedals, while your left does nothing, unless you're operating a manual transmission.

Since you do these activities most every day, these muscles are used over and over again, while others—like your left leg when driving—are hardly ever worked. You can imagine how the stronger muscles on one side of your body—with little counterbalancing resistance from the weaker ones on the other side—can pull your spine, hips, and other joints slightly out of alignment.

The same thing can happen with your forward and backward movements. Many people tend to lean forward more than backward for activities such as driving, reading, mowing the lawn, woodwork, crafts, playing games, and, of course, working at the computer. You lift heavy items by leaning forward, not backward. For sports such as skiing, running, cycling, soccer, and baseball, you're almost always leaning forward.

If you're not performing backward-type stretches and exercises to counteract these "bending forward" habits, the muscles in the front of your body will become stronger and shorter, while the muscles in the back may weaken and stretch out. Again, when the front of your body is much stronger than the back, you can imagine how such unbalanced forces can subtly distort the natural curve of your spine.

There are many more examples of how we use our muscles unevenly. You may prop a telephone on one ear while doing other tasks, using just one side of your neck. Carrying a heavy purse, laptop bag, or backpack on one shoulder may cause you to lean to one side to support the weight while sticking your hip out on the other side to counterbalance it.

A similar thing happens if you have young children or grandchildren and carry them on one hip. You jut out that hip to support the extra weight—without copying the action on the opposite side.

Another example: If you have a wallet or cell phone in your back pocket all the time, it tends to tilt your hip and the rest of your body to one side whenever you're sitting.

The result of all this uneven body use is that certain parts of the body grow strong while other parts weaken, creating a literal tug of war—where both sides lose.

Common Muscle Imbalance Examples

One of the most common examples of a muscle imbalance that causes back pain occurs in many people today who work in sedentary positions. We call it "forward-tipped pelvis." All that sitting tightens the hip flexors (fronts of hips). Meanwhile, the stomach (abdominal), hamstring, and buttock muscles become weak from being underused.

Forward-Tipped Pelvis

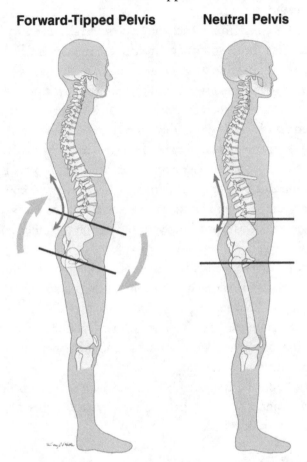

Figure 1: Forward-tipped pelvis versus neutral pelvis

The tight muscles pull the pelvis down and forward, creating an excessive curve in the lower torso and causing the abdomen to protrude forward. The resulting pressure on the lower spine can eventually cause dysfunction and injury, such as sciatica, a herniated disc, or a muscle spasm.

Another common muscle imbalance is one we like to call "forward head and shoulders."

Forward Head & Neck

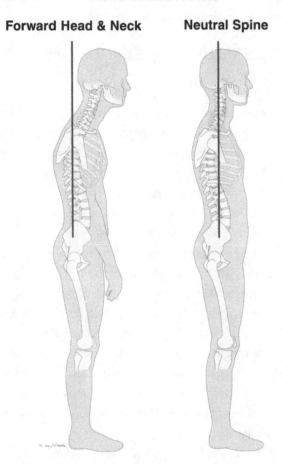

Figure 2: Forward head and neck versus neutral spine

This occurs frequently because people spend so much time hunched over computers, steering wheels, office desks, stoves—almost every activity we do requires us to lean forward.

This causes the muscles in the chest and at the base of the neck to tighten up, while the muscles in the upper back and shoulders weaken and stretch out, putting pressure on the upper spine and causing upper back and neck pain.

There are other common muscle imbalances, but perhaps you

can begin to see how our everyday routines work our muscles unevenly, create bad posture, and eventually lead to pain.

Your Muscle Strength: Use It or Lose It

The body is truly an amazing machine. The more you work it, the stronger it gets. In contrast, if you drive your car for thousands of miles, it's not going to drive any faster or get better gas mileage. If you play your upright piano for years, it's never going to grow into a grand piano. The human body, on the other hand, responds to work by becoming stronger and more efficient—especially in the muscles.

As you go about your daily routine, using one hand, arm, or leg more than the other, that part of the body becomes stronger. Imagine if you lifted weights with only your left arm for several months and did very little with your right arm. Pretty soon, you would notice a definite difference between the two.

When you exercise or use a muscle, the fibers are stimulated, stressed, or slightly "damaged." This is why you may feel sore after a particular activity. During rest, the body repairs the muscle, building it back up to withstand similar work in the future. The fascinating thing is that the body goes the extra mile in reconstruction, building the muscle up stronger than it was before, so you can handle the same activity with greater ease.

However, the opposite also is true: When you don't work a muscle, it not only doesn't grow stronger, it actually grows weaker, sort of like a basketball that isn't inflated regularly. If you've ever had an operation on one leg or arm and had to build the muscles back up again, you know this fact well!

Or, if you've ever been confined to bed for a week or two due to a medical condition, you'll remember how wobbly you felt when you tried to get up again. This is because your muscles had already started to weaken from inactivity.

So, how do these uneven muscles result in a tug-of-war inside your body?

Striving for Balance

When we think of balance, we often imagine two things working in opposition to one another. We may visualize two children on a teeter-totter, for instance, or the two ropes that lift and lower a flag on a pulley. Muscles work much the same way—in twos. In order for you to be able to move forward and back and side to side, each muscle needs a partner muscle to pull the opposite way.

If you bend your elbow to touch your neck, your biceps (the muscles on the front of the upper arm) pull, or contract and shorten, and the triceps (the muscles on the back of the upper arm) relax and go into a stretched position. If you didn't have the triceps muscles to pull your arm back out, it would remain bent. Fortunately, when you're ready, the triceps contract, while the biceps relax to straighten your arm again. This is why it's so important to keep both muscles in an opposing muscle group balanced.

I'm not saying here that both muscles need to be of equal strength, as some muscles are naturally designed to be stronger than others.

Rather, each muscle should maintain the state of strength and flexibility that keeps the nearby joints functioning optimally. This allows you to move easily in all directions in the way the body was designed to move.

When it comes to eliminating and preventing back pain, the goal isn't necessarily to have muscles as strong and flexible as possible— though that certainly helps. The goal, as we said in Chapter 5, is balance: Your muscle pairs need balanced strength and flexibility to support your body height and weight and allow for normal movement.

Unfortunately, for most of us, keeping all the muscle pairs equally balanced is a tall order. Not only do we suffer from working some too much and others too little, we suffer from *stretching* some too much and others too little. But the even bigger challenge is that most people aren't even aware of this. While this basic understanding of how our bodies work should be common knowledge, it isn't, and that's why so many people struggle with nagging aches and pains.

"I Can't Touch My Toes Anymore!"

Many of us, as we get older, become less flexible. When we were children we could probably touch our toes, do somersaults, and even perform splits. But as we get older, our muscles seem to tighten up like boards. You may be surprised to hear that age isn't the main culprit.

A muscle's natural reaction is to contract. Just like a roly-poly bug that curls up when you touch it, the muscle—when you ask it to work—will tighten.

Think of what happens when you touch a hot burner by mistake. The muscle contracts to pull your hand away, sometimes before you even realize what's happened.

Similarly, when you perform an activity, the muscle contracts to help you perform it. That means for every activity you do, some muscle, somewhere, is pulling or contracting. Do the activity frequently and for extended periods of time, and the muscle is required to stay in that short, contracted state.

If the muscle is stretched during a resting and healing period, it most likely will return to its relaxed, elongated, and more flexible state. (This is why most fitness trainers, like me, recommend stretching after exercising, to elongate the muscle again after it's been tightened from physical activity.) If it's not stretched, it will stay tight, and at the end of the healing process, it will remain a little shorter than it was before.

For most of us who do certain activities over and over again, but fail to adopt a regular stretching routine, this is how we lose flexibility.

Gradually, our muscles get so used to being in a contracted, tightened state that they tend to stay that way. Suddenly, we can no longer touch our toes—or for some folks, even our knees!

Muscle Flexibility: Stretch It or Lose It

If you're a woman who wears high heels, most likely you've heard the warnings: Wear them too much and the muscles in the backs of your lower legs—the calf muscles—will shorten. And if you haven't, here it is now: Wearing high heels is asking for problems, and it's one of the worst things you can do to your feet and body. You can visualize this effect.

Just imagine your calf muscle as a rubber band that extends from the back of your knee to your heel. When you wear high heels, the rubber band contracts (or gets shorter) to accommodate the shorter distance between your heel and your knee. Over time—particularly if you wear these shoes up to eight hours a day, five days a week—the muscle adapts to this shorter position, so that when you take the high heels off, you feel a pull as the calf muscle tries to lengthen again to set your heel on the floor.

The same thing can happen to the muscles in the backs of your thighs, called the hamstrings. Visually, you can imagine the hamstring "rubber band" at a certain length when you're standing. What happens when you sit down? The rubber band—in this case, the muscle in the back of the leg—shortens to allow you to sit.

If you sit too much, the muscle will adapt itself to that position as normal and become permanently shortened, again, reducing your flexibility and causing pain when you stand or need to bend over. This shortening of the muscles happens throughout the body, with any muscle that is required to remain in a shortened position for a long time—and is stretched too little.

Lack of stretching and overwork of muscles are a couple of reasons why we lose flexibility. But there is another reason, which you never hear health care professionals talk about: excess fibrin. A more common term for it is "scar tissue." I'll talk more about fibrin in Chapter 8, but for now, understand that when you work a muscle, some of the fibers are damaged. This is a good thing, because when the body goes into repair mode, it typically builds the muscle back stronger than it was before.

However, part of that rebuilding process involves producing fibrin, or "scar tissue," which forms a sort of latticework on which the body can build new tissue. (Picture the crisscross framework on a building undergoing remodeling.) To provide maximum structural integrity for your injured tissues and joints, fibrin is a naturally stiff and inflexible material. The more fibrin that builds up in your body, the more inflexible you become.

Typically, once the repair work is finished, a special group of enzymes called proteolytic enzymes come in to complete the job by breaking down the fibrin and whisking it away. Unfortunately, as we get older, our bodies don't produce as much of these critical enzymes as when we were younger. Without these enzymes doing the cleanup job, fibrin builds up in our connecting tissues. This is why, when you turn 40, 50, or 60, you begin to feel stiff all over and less springy than when you were younger.

You can see how our tug-of-war is getting worse. Not only is it going on between strong versus weak muscle pairs, it's happening between flexible versus inflexible muscle pairs. And guess what's in the middle of the battle? Your spine—specifically your neck, back, and hips.

Watch these videos to learn more about
muscle imbalances and how to correct them:
www.losethebackpain.com/muscleimbalances

Chapter 15 contains further information about identifying and treating muscle imbalances.

Trigger Points

Muscle imbalances are not the only physical causes of back pain. Another source is something known as trigger points, or "knots," in one or more of your muscles.

When you use your muscles, your body tells them to contract. Long, hair-like muscle fibers lock together, shorten, and draw in. For example, when you lift your coffee cup, muscle fibers in your bicep contract, allowing your arm to lift. When you're done lifting, your body tells these muscle fibers to relax. The fibers "unlock" and allow your muscle to elongate.

When a muscle is overworked (contracted "too much"), it may simply radiate pain, but oftentimes a knot will also develop. (In the case of a tendon or ligament, inflammation or injury may occur.) These knots are really small tangles in the fibers of your muscles.

If you've ever had a massage, you're probably familiar with this. Knots are tender, feel hard to the touch, and can require a lot of pressure to release. If you think of the muscle as a length of hair—since muscles are made of up fibers similar to hair strands—a normal muscle would look like healthy, combed hair, whereas a muscle suffering from a knot would look like you took the hair and twisted it.

This knot slows blood flow through the muscle, causing several problems. First, the waste products produced by your muscle cells aren't removed quickly, so they settle into the fibers.

Second, the cells in those areas aren't getting as much oxygen as they're used to getting—so they're mildly oxygen deprived.

Third, your blood transports the fuel that powers the "unlocking" mechanism within those last few muscle fibers that are "stuck" together. Without ample blood circulation, these muscle fibers never unlock. This creates a vicious self-reinforcing cycle where a knot causes slow blood circulation, which prevents the knot from releasing itself, which causes the knot to persist even further. (This is a classic situation of your blood circulation moving "too slow" in that specific part of your body.)

These three conditions combine to cause inflammation, tenderness, and pain in that part of the muscle. The result is a trigger point, or what most people think of as a knot, in their muscle.

It's also important to note that trigger points can develop in tendons, and because tendons are so much less vascular, meaning they get so much less blood flow, they often are much harder to treat effectively.

Videos to help you identify and learn more
about trigger points are available at
www.losethebackpain.com/triggerpoints

Physical Dysfunctions and Conditions

A physical dysfunction occurs when your body posture and/or mechanics are no longer optimal, or "normal," and are now creating excessive wear and tear on your muscles, ligaments, bones, and joints. This can show up simply as pain, or it can develop into a medical condition, such as scoliosis, a joint condition, disc herniation, and more.

Imagine a puppet. If you pull one string up tight and leave the others loose, the body will change posture. The same is true of your muscles. The tighter, shorter ones will pull your body out of its normal position and the result will be a curved or crooked posture.

This is what happens to our bodies when the muscles are out of balance. The changes may be subtle, but we're walking around in twisted ways and, eventually, we'll experience pain and/or suffer an outright condition, such as a herniated disc or sciatica. Vertebrae are pulled to the right or left, straining the spine. Hips are pitched forward or backward, forcing the lower back into an unnatural position. Shoulders round, pulling on the upper back and neck. These joints and bones are then forced to move every day in these strange, tilted positions.

When you have a physical dysfunction, your body will try to compensate. In other words, it "works around" whatever the dysfunction is in order to do what you want it to do, whether that be a particular exercise or a particular task. For example, if you sit for many hours of the day (like many people do), your hip flexors—those muscles on the front of your hips that pull your knees up—become short and tight. This tightness can "pull" the top of the pelvis on one or both sides downward, which creates excessive curvature in your lower back. Then you have constant strain placed on the muscles of the lower back, but that's nothing compared to the uneven compression placed on your discs as a result of the excess curvature.

This is just one example of how physical dysfunctions develop and wreak havoc on our bodies. As someone with back, neck, or sciatic pain, it is critical that you understand this process, as it holds the key to you getting lasting relief and also knowing how to prevent or better deal with future flare-ups.

How Physical Dysfunctions Create "Conditions" and Pain

If you regularly carry a wallet, cell phone, or other object in your pants pocket, try the following exercise. Put on a pair of fairly snug-fitting jeans that have a back pocket and sit in a chair. Notice your body position. Then stand up, put the wallet or cell phone in the back pocket and sit back down again. See how your body position shifts ever so slightly? The hip on the same side as the wallet or phone will rise up a little bit, and your shoulders and neck will adapt to compensate. This is the same thing your body does when lifting a heavy bag, though the effect is a bit subtler.

Here's another demonstration you should do in front of a full-length mirror or with a friend who can take a photograph of you. Stand with your side to the mirror (or camera). Next, place your hands on your hips. Notice how your index finger and thumb rest on your hips.

If you were to put a carpenter's bubble level on the area covered by your index finger and thumb, would you be "level"? Ideally, you want to be. But if your index finger and thumb lean toward the front of your body, your hips lean too far forward. This puts you at much greater risk for back pain. Similarly, if your finger and index finger lean toward the back of your body, your hips lean too far backward, which also can lead to back pain.

Or try this. Face the mirror, or the camera, with your hands at your sides and then stand to the side. Look at yourself in the mirror or in the photos. Do your fingers rest on the side of your leg or do they rest more toward the front, on the big leg muscles called the quadriceps?

If someone looking at the front of your body can see your knuckles, this is a problem. The correct position is for your hands and knuckles to rest at the sides of your body—clearly visible to someone to your right or left, but not to someone who is facing you.

If your hands rest in the forward-rotated position, also known as "forward-rolled shoulders," it means many of the muscles in the front of the upper body are much shorter and tighter (not always, but typically stronger) than the corresponding muscles in the back. People who spend a lot of time driving and have to reach for the steering wheel, or who sit in front of a computer where the keyboard is too far away, often show this type of imbalanced pattern.

The Slippery Slope Toward Back Pain

When a physical condition isn't corrected, the body starts to break down. Usually the result is pain, which can exist on its own without signaling any particular condition. However, conditions also arise as a result of the same lengthy wear and tear.

Tight muscles can pull the vertebrae out of alignment, pinching a nerve or creating a herniated disc. Physical dysfunctions can pressure joints and, over time, stress them to the maximum until they develop inflammation and injury. Overworked muscles can go into spasm, causing pain and forcing the body into physical dysfunction.

The pain from these conditions is often triggered by some sort of activity, such as heavy lifting, gardening, cleaning, or sports. Suddenly there is pain, as the result of a muscle spasm, strain, or pull, or by a pinched nerve or inflamed joint.

That's why most people believe they have "thrown out" their backs or suffered the injury because of a singular occurrence. The condition shows up immediately after the activity, so the belief is that the activity caused the condition. However, this is rarely the case. The activity may have triggered the pain, but it was the long months or years of uneven muscle use that actually created the condition that made the pain possible.

Back Pain Type #1:
Nerve-Based Back Pain

Once the physical dysfunction and/or condition exists, pain can be triggered suddenly and without warning at any time. When you have a muscle or bone that is a hair's length away from a nerve, it doesn't take much for either of them to intrude on the nerve's space—irritating it and causing you nerve-based back pain.

Incidentally, one of the main reasons so many back treatments fail, work only temporarily, or have inconsistent results is because most treatment approaches focus on the latter steps of this process. There are many ways to make pain go away temporarily, but all such relief measures don't address the underlying causes of the pain.

For example, surgery may claim to "correct a herniated disc," but it does nothing to address the physical dysfunctions and muscle imbalances that caused the disc to herniate in the first place. This is why many who have back surgery end up having repeat back surgery. One disc gets "fixed," only to have another become damaged a year or two later as a result of the same muscle imbalances that were never corrected. And that's assuming the disc was really what caused the pain to begin with.

Rather than get a new bucket to catch water leaking from a roof, it makes a lot more sense to just fix the hole in the roof. The same can be said for back pain. Find the source of the problem and all the "downstream" issues end up disappearing on their own—including the pain!

Back Pain Type #2:
Tissue-Based Back Pain

When a physical dysfunction or condition persists uncorrected, the various tissues in your body—namely your muscles, tendons, and ligaments—get overworked incredibly quickly. Normally, these tissues are strained only when you use them. Under these kinds of conditions, your soft tissues can tolerate enormous usage completely pain free.

But if you have a physical dysfunction, you're actually straining those soft tissues virtually every second of your waking day.

For example, if your hips are misaligned due to a muscle imbalance or trigger point, the muscles surrounding your misaligned hips get overworked and abused. If you're sitting in a chair under these conditions, your muscles, tendons, and ligaments have to work overtime to compensate for your physical dysfunction. This quickly becomes excess usage (the "too much" problem we mentioned previously) and your body rebels by making you feel pain.

Why Didn't My Doctor Tell Me About This?

You may be wondering why your doctor never told you about muscle imbalances; trigger points; the excess, deficiency, and stagnation; and the mind-body-diet concepts. Certainly, he or she is an educated person. Do doctors not know about them? And how can that be?

The fact is, in the United States, and most other "modern" countries, medical schools tend to focus on treating the symptoms, and the solutions they favor usually include pharmaceuticals or surgery.

If you suffer a heart attack, for instance, because of a blocked artery, doctors will focus on opening that artery (either with surgery or medication) and give little attention to why the artery became blocked in the first place. Then, to help you avoid another blocked artery, they'll prescribe drugs, rather than investigate the "why" behind your condition.

Most of our medical professionals work very hard for their credentials, and they tend to work equally as hard in their practices. It takes an enormous amount of time and effort just to stay current with all the advances in the medical world, including new drugs, new treatments, and new technologies.

Unfortunately, insurance companies put enormous time-management pressures on doctors. They only have a few minutes to make you feel better—and a few minutes are nowhere near enough to identify the underlying causes of your pain, let alone develop a comprehensive treatment plan.

At the same time, pharmaceutical companies are creating billions of dollars in profit each year so rather than a focus on prevention it's on how to sell more drugs and what new drugs can be developed.

And while the typical doctor's visit isn't long enough to really solve a back pain problem, it is long enough to prescribe the latest and greatest pill—a pill that may temporarily reduce pain but doesn't get rid of the underlying causes of the pain, and that is usually not without serious negative side effects.

Even if your doctor orders diagnostic tests such as an MRI or X-ray, these can only identify the presence of a specific condition, such as a herniated disc, not its cause.

Simply treating the condition only sets up a vicious cycle. When the underlying causes of back pain aren't addressed, you end up right back in the doctor's office a few months later with the exact same problem you had previously. And the whole process repeats itself.

The drug companies continue to make money with each back pain episode you experience. In a misguided attempt to save money, insurance companies feel like they've succeeded because they've kept doctors' visits very brief—so they can pay them less.

Of course, when you don't actually solve what's causing your back pain, you end up having to go back to your doctor repeatedly. This costs insurance companies more in the long run, but they're so used to thinking about short-term profits they often don't look at it from any other perspective.

Fortunately for you, there are other approaches to resolving back pain that do not rely on surgery or potentially harmful medications.

Keep in mind that muscle imbalances and trigger points are technically not diseases. Most doctors and the medical schools that train them focus only on eliminating diseases. And since most forms of back pain technically aren't diseases, many medical doctors aren't familiar with these alternative approaches.

It's Not *Your* Fault

If you're thinking, "What's the matter with me? Why didn't I notice this was happening?," stop. Don't be hard on yourself. You didn't notice because your body made the changes without you being aware of them. You may have experienced some aches and pains, but who hasn't, right? Besides, most of us are hard-pressed to find the time to really focus on our health until our bodies literally demand it.

It isn't your fault that you've suffered back pain. The good news is now that you're taking a proactive approach to your condition, you're going to learn what you need to know to take better care of your own body, get rid of the pain, and finally get your life back. This knowledge will last the rest of your life, helping you make adjustments when you need to, so you'll reduce your chances of ever having to experience back pain again.

Remember, we all have these imbalances, and the sooner you identify and address them, the sooner you'll be on your way to freedom from pain. Later in this book, I'll teach you exactly how you can do just that.

Your Mind and Your Diet:
Two Other Potential Sources of Back Pain

While problems in the body tend to be the ones most doctors and health care professionals focus on, the mind and diet play a much bigger role than most realize. In fact, I personally feel, and more and more research is suggesting, that these other areas may be keys to improving back pain. It's quite easy to have issues with "too much," "too little," and blood circulation or body energy that's "too slow" because of your emotional and dietary life. We'll cover these areas in detail in the next two chapters.

Still in pain? My free "Stuck in Pain" video series can help! Watch it at: **www.losethebackpain.com/stillinpain**

CHAPTER 7

THE MIND: HOW EMOTIONS CAUSE PHYSICAL PAIN

Know, then, whatever cheerful and serene
supports the mind supports the body, too.
John Armstrong

Most of us have been conditioned to believe that if we feel pain, something is wrong with our bodies. Particularly with back pain, we assume we've pulled a muscle, herniated a disc, or suffered some other injury or condition that's causing discomfort.

Of course, this may be the case. But what we may not realize is that sometimes the hidden cause of physical pain can have emotional origins. We can experience too much stress, anxiety, trauma, sadness, anger, and emotional pain, and too little relaxation, stress relief, joy, fun, security, and calm.

All of us suffer physically when our emotional lives are in upheaval. We often experience physical symptoms of pain or discomfort because of anger, fear, anxiety, sadness, or other negative emotions. These types of emotional stressors don't need to be catastrophic or provoke mental illness to trigger a chain of events leading to back pain.

It's important to recognize that in these cases, the pain is not imaginary or "in your head." Instead, the triggering cause can be an emotional issue that, if left unchecked, can create physical conditions in your body that make it highly susceptible to pain—especially back pain.

In fact, an extensive study conducted by Stanford University on more than 3,000 employees at the Boeing Corporation found that emotions and psychological factors were the biggest indicators of back pain.

How Emotions Act on the Body

The mind is inextricably connected to the body. You have only to imagine stepping off a bridge to feel your stomach fly up into your throat and your muscles tense. This mental thought can trigger a chain of physical reactions, including dramatic fluctuations in blood pressure, breathing rates, oxygen levels, and more.

Just thinking about a stressful event can cause all this!

So you can see the effect your mind can have on your body, particularly if you're thinking stressful thoughts many times throughout the day. Your muscles tighten and, if you remember from the last chapter, tight muscles cause problems. They inhibit circulation, constricting blood vessels so the blood doesn't flow through your body like it should and creating muscle imbalances.

Without adequate blood flow, the cells in your body become slightly oxygen deprived. Toxins and waste aren't cleaned out as efficiently as they should be and can build up in certain parts of your body, creating or reactivating trigger points. These knots are often painful to the touch and, in some cases, can cause muscles to spasm or "lock up," which can pull your spinal column out of align-ment—pinching nerves and causing nerve-based back pain.

If you doubt the effects the mind can have on the body, let me tell you about a study that was done in Finland. Autopsies were performed on people who had died from non-back-pain-related causes but had reported suffering from back pain while alive. Researchers were shocked to find that the average person with back pain had two arteries to the spine completely blocked off. And remember, without fresh blood supplying oxygen and nutrients, it's nearly impossible to heal.

Stress also alters your breathing. Typically, when you're anxious or upset, your breath becomes shallow, reducing oxygen flow to the whole body. Oxygen and nutrients don't circulate at optimum levels, again contributing to the buildup of toxins. Stress also can release hormones, such as adrenaline, which can trigger chronic tension and inflammation in your muscles, ligaments, and tendons. Without adequate blood flow to remove these hormones from the body, they can linger longer than usual and create more damage.

That all these changes have a debilitating effect on the back is no surprise. Which muscles do you tend to tense most when you're anxious? Shoulders usually come first, directly affecting the spine. The jaw, stomach, and lower back also are very common areas. It's no wonder the back and head are some of the first parts of the body to suffer from stress.

Other Ways Emotions Affect Health

Negative emotions can have other detrimental effects on our health—effects that can make back pain worse.

Think about an emotionally distressing episode in your life. You probably slept too little, depriving your body of its primary healing time. Maybe your diet went off kilter somehow, so you either lost your appetite and ate too little or reverted to eating too many highly processed, low-nutrient foods. You might have skipped your usual exercise routine, moving your body too little and sitting too much. People around you may have commented on your increased irritability, or maybe you blew up at someone and later regretted it.

All these occasions are like dominoes stacked up against your health and well-being. Too little sleep, exercise, and calm, along with too much anxiety, bad foods, and inactivity all can have profound effects on your body. Back pain, neck pain, headaches, jaw pain, and joint soreness are all just around the corner.

What makes this especially difficult is that the emotional component of any painful condition often is ignored. Somehow we're conditioned to believe that any physical manifestation of our feelings is a sign of weakness or some mental problem.

This is, of course, as silly as thinking that when someone yells "Boo!" and startles your mind, it's abnormal if your heart races. On the contrary, it's quite typical to have a mental burden impact your physical body.

As a society, we accept that being diagnosed with cancer or suffering a heart attack—even having a baby—can cause emotions like depression, anger, and even guilt.

What we don't recognize as easily is that the communication works both ways—from mind to body and from body to mind. Science has proven that the brain's messengers (neurotransmitters) communicate information in the brain and throughout the body. Since the mind itself operates on physical and chemical reactions, why wouldn't emotions, which are communicated in physical ways inside the body, have very physical outcomes?

The truth is that our thoughts and emotions, and how we handle them, all have a very large effect on our everyday health and well-being. During periods of stress, they certainly cause or exacerbate physical discomfort or injury.

How Do You Handle Emotions?

How we handle our emotions determines how they will affect us physically. It's an unfortunate thing that as children we're rarely taught how to deal with our feelings. While we were learning all about reading, writing, math, and science—unless our parents were especially gifted in teaching us—we learned very little about the art of mastering our own emotions.

If we were angry and blew up, most likely we were sent to our rooms, or if we were in school, to the principal's office. If we were depressed, many times we were told to snap out of it or to stop feeling sorry for ourselves.

As teens, we were more likely to get lectures and lose privileges than have honest conversations about how we were feeling.

Those of us fortunate enough to have received some instruction along the way may have avoided the aches and pains that come from raging emotions.

But for many of us, we never learned the art of expressing ourselves without hurting others, or how journaling, meditating, or "walking off" steam are healthier approaches to dealing with emotions like anger, resentment, or sadness.

Some of us may not even realize when a powerful emotion has taken hold of us. We just react by yelling, hitting things, or turning to self-destructive habits like alcohol or drug use. Others grew up learning to be nice and to refrain from hurting others' feelings, repressing emotions until they erupted into medical conditions.

Psychology has shown us that, by far, the most dangerous way to handle emotions is to deny or repress them. If we don't learn to express them (in healthy ways), they stay in our bodies, sometimes for years, steadily wearing away our resistance to their destructive powers.

Learning to properly express and deal with our emotions is one of the best things we can do for our overall health, and especially for back pain.

Destructive Emotions

Level 1: Everyday Stress

When we consider the effects emotions can have on our systems, we can imagine four different levels of severity. Level one is the everyday stress we're all subjected to, especially with today's fast-paced lifestyle. The morning commute, the demands of the job, watching over our children, managing our relationships, and dealing with daily crises like no milk, flat tires, forgotten lunches, scraped knees, visiting relatives, broken sinks, unpaid bills, and sick cats.

Most of us handle these types of stressors fairly well, but there's no doubt that unless we are consciously aware of the tension they can cause, they still can affect our bodies negatively. Many people will "hold" tension in the shoulders by clenching the muscles, forgetting to "let go" of the stress.

When these muscles are locked up for long periods of time, blood flow slows down and the unlocking mechanism doesn't work. The resulting trigger point or knot can be the beginning of pain. If we don't take the time to unwind, burn off stress through exercise, or relax when the day is over, we may carry that tension to bed, where it will disrupt sleep and interrupt the healing process the body normally conducts at night.

Little stresses can pile up until the body reaches a tipping point and triggers pain or is unable to keep you from getting rid of it.

Level 2: Stressful Occurrences

In addition to the stress in our everyday lives, we can sometimes experience events that aren't necessarily out of the ordinary, but that ratchet up stress levels nonetheless.

A car accident, even if we're not hurt, can rattle us and cause tension that lasts for hours. A promotion or demotion at work can create weeks of anxiety as we adapt to the new position. If one of our children is struggling in school, we may spend hours worrying, contacting teachers, and trying to set up help for the child.

Unexpected expenses, such as a house repair when we don't have the money for it, can elevate our stress levels. Strained relationships with our spouses or other relatives can stir our stomachs for months.

These events could be considered "level 2" stressors—those that aren't part of our normal day-to-day existence but can disrupt our regular routines. Again, how we deal with them is more important than the events themselves. If we feel confident that we can handle them and take gradual steps to do so, we'll feel much better than if we feel victimized ("Why me?") or incapable of solving the problems.

Like level 1 stressors, level 2 stressors can constrict blood flow (so it moves "too slowly" through the body), creating trigger points or knots and, ultimately, back pain. The difference is that level 2 stressors can accelerate the process so that back pain results much more quickly and/ or becomes more severe.

Level 3: Major Life Events

Many of us have heard about the "top five" stressors in life. Usually, these are:

1.   Death
2.   Job change
3.   Marriage
4.   Divorce
5.   Personal injury

Experiencing any of these events puts a heavy load on your system. This is when you must call on all your resources for help: family and friends, support groups, counselors, doctors, massage therapists, personal trainers, and more.

No matter how you look at it, these events are going to affect you both physically and emotionally. The key is to put in place all the support you can so that you can recover as quickly as possible.

Maintaining a healthy diet, exercising regularly, and talking or journaling about your feelings all can help you cope.

One thing we often run up against in these situations is the resistance to taking care of ourselves. It's not that we're not capable of self-care, but that self-care has a negative connotation for us.

It's difficult to admit that we need some time off, a vacation, someone to talk to, someone to help us. We somehow believe that taking time for ourselves is selfish. After all, we have our families, our children, and our jobs to think about. Too often, we dive right back into our usual routines without taking the time to process and reflect on the situation that has just affected us so profoundly.

If you suffer a personal injury, such as a broken leg, severed limb, or heart attack, you're forced to remain in the hospital for a certain length of time. Your body requires that you be still and rest in order to properly recover. We accept this without question.

Yet, we're reluctant to believe that our minds and emotions need similar recovery time after, say, a death in the family or a divorce. It doesn't make any sense. Rest and recovery is necessary after any trauma—whether the trauma is physical or emotional in nature.

Taking time in these instances to get away for a while, reflect, journal, and provide ourselves proper care goes a long way toward helping us avoid physical pain in the future.

Level 4: Buried Emotions—The Most Destructive Kind

At level four are the most destructive emotions of all—those that are repressed or buried. Most often, these come about as a result of trauma, either in our childhood or adulthood, that we never completely understood or processed. Childhood abuse and abandonment, rape, and being witness to a murder or other violence are all examples of this type of trauma. Wartime events fall under this category; incidents can haunt soldiers for years. These experiences have huge, catastrophic effects on our minds and our bodies and, if not processed thoroughly, can lodge themselves inside us where they will continue to hurt us for years to come.

Repressed emotions, like anger, anxiety, and fear, can tighten muscles, reducing blood flow to areas such as the back and the neck—leading to back pain. Many times, this is an unconscious reaction to the old trauma, and the person is not even aware of the emotion causing the pain.

In the 1970s, Dr. John Sarno, a professor at the New York University School of Medicine, first identified this emotionally caused form of back pain, called tension myositis syndrome (TMS).

According to Dr. Sarno, TMS doesn't respond to normal back pain treatments; instead, it keeps coming back because the underlying cause is repressed emotions.

The key to solving this type of back pain is for the patient to become aware of the sometimes "hidden" emotions causing it. Dr. Sarno and other doctors advise patients to "think psychological."

For individuals who have gone through the usual tests and found no physical problems causing their pain, this technique can be especially helpful. In other words, when the pain strikes, instead of thinking about the part of the body that must be damaged ("Oh, there goes my herniated disc" or "Ouch, that muscle is getting me again"), the patient is told to understand that the body is perfectly fine and to think about what emotion could be at the root of the pain.

Are you feeling particularly alone right now in your life? Do you feel a lack of support? Is there some pain in the past that could be causing you trouble? If you were to ask the pain where it comes from, what would it say? (It may be wise to do this sort of probing with a licensed psychologist.)

Taking the time to do some thinking about the emotions that could be causing your pain could be the key to your cure. Oftentimes, simply acknowledging the psychological aspect of the pain and identifying the offending emotion can diminish its power within days.

Emotions and Back Pain: The Vicious Cycle

Even if back pain is caused by physical factors, emotions can delay recovery. For example, many people who suffer- from back pain caused by physical reasons often feel very frustrated by the experience. Frustration is an emotional stressor—which as you may have guessed, can slow blood flow and make preexisting back pain even worse. This then doubles the frustration level, and the whole cycle repeats itself.

Negative emotions feed into the pain. This is another reason why it's so important to solve your back pain as quickly as possible—so the pain will not become chronic. If we try to go about "life as usual," we'll probably fail to give our bodies (and minds) the attention they need to heal properly, and then we'll be saddled with pain for weeks, months, even years.

This is a dangerous situation because it can be much harder to fix chronic pain than it is to fix pain that has existed for only a short time. Once chronic pain takes hold, it becomes much more difficult to fend off emotions like frustration and anxiety, which only make the pain hang around longer.

It doesn't help that so often our medical community suggests drugs or surgery for back pain symptoms. These "solutions" can cause people stress, anxiety, and fear, and when they don't cure the problem, they've actually made it worse by ratcheting up the anxiety surrounding the whole situation.

So What Can I Do?

In the next section of this book, we'll cover methods you can use TO address back pain caused by some mental or emotional burden. But first, let's look at the final potential source of back pain—your diet.

CHAPTER 8

THE DIET:
HOW DIETARY
IMBALANCES
CAUSE PAIN

Life is not merely to be alive, but to be well.
Marcus Valerius Martial

So far we have discussed how back pain is caused by having too much of something, too little of something, or blood circulation that's too slow. These three things can occur as a result of problems in your physical body, mind, and/or diet. In this chapter, we're going to discuss diet—particularly, how food and water can either make your back pain better or worse.

Most of us, on a daily basis, eat too much of foods that increase the likelihood of back pain, and too little of what prevents it. The effects can often slow down the digestive system, blood flow, or transportation of waste. What you may not realize is that these secondary effects can have a direct effect on back pain.

For most people, this concept comes as a surprise. "My back hurts," they say. "How in the world is that related to what I eat?"

Let me explain.

Your body depends on food and water for energy, healing, cleansing, and your very survival. These are the only things your body has to help it perform optimally.

Imagine if you "fed" your car something other than gas. What if the fuel was contaminated with dirt, foreign chemicals, or even chocolate chips? You may not notice the effects immediately, but soon you'd hear the telltale clicking and coughing of mechanical parts grinding down, sticking together, and losing force and propulsion. Your car might fail to start or lose power going uphill. If you fix the problem, clean out the engine, replace a few parts, and add clean fuel, you'll probably go on all right. But what if you kept filling the car with the same junk? Surely you wouldn't expect it to keep performing?

Yet we do this very thing to our bodies, which are also machines, just of the organic variety. We don't feed them enough, feed them too much, or stuff them with things that only clog up our internal parts. You may have chuckled at the idea of car fuel contaminated with chocolate chips, but many of the things you ingest every day are just as foreign to your body as chocolate chips would be to your gas tank!

I'm not just talking about eating "healthy" here, to lose weight, for instance, or to trim unwanted belly fat to relieve pressure from your back. Of course, that may help, but it's only part of the story.

Most people think of food in terms of "healthiness"—healthful food versus junk food, for example. You may think of foods that make you fat as unhealthful and foods that keep your body lean and strong as healthful.

While conceptually this thinking is mostly correct, there's an entirely different way to look at food that's relevant for back pain. Instead of the traditional notion of eating healthful versus unhealthful foods, you also want to think of foods in terms of their ability to enhance or reduce pain.

It's true. Certain types of foods make your body more sensitive to pain and can increase the severity of it—especially back pain. Other foods actually reduce pain levels and decrease your ability to notice them.

Why People Feel Pain

Before we get into how food can cause or keep you in pain, it helps to have a basic understanding of how pain works. Like everything in the body, it's a physical and chemical response, governed by nerve fibers that we can imagine as telephone wires. Throughout the body we have strings of these nerve fibers, much like the thousands of telephone wires that connect various parts of the country. At one end of a single fiber is a pain receptor, which we can think of as the phone in your house, and at the other end is the receiver—the "operator"—set up in the spinal cord.

When the body senses something is wrong, the nerve endings, or receptors, send a message. The message travels as an electronic signal along the nerve fibers to the spinal cord. There, either the "operator" transmits the message to the brain—in which case you feel the pain— or the "operator" fails to send the message and you don't feel the pain. Only if and when the signal reaches the brain are you consciously aware of it.

As you already know, all pain isn't the same. There are different types. One is in reaction to an injury, like a broken bone, burnt finger, or tissues eroded by cancer.

Another is caused by abnormalities in the nerves, spinal cord, or brain, and is usually felt as a burning, tingling, shooting, or electric sensation.

There is acute pain, which is normally very sharp but resolves quickly when the problem is solved.

Finally, there is chronic pain, which goes on and on for a long time. Chronic pain can be caused by ongoing tissue damage, or it can be a disorder in itself, where something is wrong with the pain receptors, the nerve pathways, or the spinal cord.

The main point is that pain is a physical/chemical response that can be affected by any physical or chemical changes in the body. Put contaminated fuel in your car and you will notice a change in its function. Your car may not be able to say "ouch," but you can!

Water, the First Line of Defense

When talking about diet, water often is ignored. Yet it should be the first item on the list. Water is the lifeblood of our existence, second only to air. Without it, we wouldn't survive much longer than three or so days. It cleans out toxins, hydrates tissues and organs, regulates body temperature, and supplies oxygen, which is involved in nearly all chemical processes in the body. And one more thing—it makes up a good portion of the spinal cord.

Picture a skeleton for a moment. Between every two vertebrae (bones that make up the spine) lies a disc, a doughnut-shaped ring much like a tire tube, which cushions the bone and acts as a shock absorber. This disc is made up of two parts: the outer ring, which is a flexible, but strong, substance filled with a gel-like material, and the inner ring, which is made up mostly of water. As we go about our daily activities, putting body weight on these discs, that water is gradually squeezed out. At night, the discs rehydrate, as long as there is enough water to supply them. The discs also can reabsorb more water whenever the spine moves—again, as long as there's water available for them to take in.

That inner water-filled ring is designed to shoulder about 75 percent of the weight load on the spine. The body's shock absorber, it's a water-filled cushion that supports you much like a waterbed. The outer ring, on the other hand, is supposed to carry only about 25 percent of the body's weight. However, when there's not enough water in the body to hydrate the discs, that inner ring deflates, forcing the outer ring to carry more weight than it should. Since the outer ring wasn't designed for this, it can signal pain, cause swelling, or even rupture—causing a herniated disc.

Suddenly we can see why drinking water can be so important to the spine. Water is, essentially, the cushioning between the vertebrae, the substance that absorbs the brunt of all our activities throughout the day. When you give the body enough water, you're essentially "inflating" those rings, increasing the support for your body weight and reducing your risk of pain. When you don't drink enough water, the rings deflate and dry out, putting more pressure on the vertebrae and outer rings.

Lack of water affects the muscles and joints, as well. You know how a grape looks when it dries out? Our bodies are similar. As the water supply goes down, our skin wrinkles and our muscles "shrink," leaving the joints to rub together more closely, which can cause pain.

In addition, without enough water, the body isn't able to flush away toxins as well. Sometimes that waste starts to accumulate in our systems, and the nerve endings register the chemical change as pain. Similar to the way you might feel alarmed if you were to discover a sewage leak in your home, your body sends out a red alert if toxins are found collecting somewhere they shouldn't be collecting.

Unfortunately, we rarely attribute the pain we feel to something as simple as a water shortage. But think about it. How much water are you really drinking during the day? And I mean water, not some other drink like soda, coffee, or juice that the body has to filter first. When was the last time you drank a full glass of water? Do you drink several throughout the day or one in the morning and maybe one late at night? Or only when you're downing pain pills?

The general recommendation is eight 8-ounce glasses a day, but it really depends on your body weight and your activity level. Someone who weighs more should be drinking more, and the more active you are, the more water your body uses. Get in the habit of taking water with you wherever you go, and strive to see your urine go to a pale yellow or clear color. It won't be that way first thing in the morning (after a night of no water) or after you take vitamins or eat a meal, but in general, if your urine is a heavy yellow, you're not getting enough water.

Try drinking it more often, and see how much it helps. It's a ridiculously simple solution and can quickly reduce certain types of back pain, as well as many other ailments, including headaches and muscle cramps.

Inflammation: The Raw Ingredient for Back Pain

Inflammation is quickly turning out to be the underlying contributor to all kinds of diseases and life-threatening medical conditions. It's behind most forms of pain, disease, and aging—even heart disease, arthritis, diabetes, and Alzheimer's and other degenerative diseases.

So what exactly is inflammation, and how is it involved in back pain?

To oversimplify, inflammation is a form of swelling within your body. One example is the redness and puffiness that happens around an injury, such as a sprained ankle or a cut finger. It's the body's natural response to any injury.

In the case of an external injury, like a cut or scrape, inflammation is visible in the red skin and swelling reactions. However, inflammation also can occur inside of us, where we're completely unaware of it—and it's this internal inflammation that's of greater concern.

Under normal circumstances, internal inflammation is a natural response to a specific problem or injury, which fades away when the problem is solved. But in today's world—in large part because of what most people eat—the body's inflammation response is perpetually active. It never dies down, putting enormous strain on organs (like the heart), muscle tissues, and nerve endings.

Incidentally, inflammation of the heart muscle exists in almost all heart attack cases. The inflammation wears out the muscle until it breaks down. The result is a heart attack.

Keep in mind that your heart is really just a muscle—a vital one to be sure, but still a muscle.

The same process can happen to the muscles and pain receptors in your back. When the inflammation level is high in these areas, your body reacts to the hostile environment by causing you back pain. This is really your body's way of saying, "This inflammation is too much for the back muscles to handle. Stop the inflammation, please!"

How Inflammation Causes Back Pain

Inflammation is involved with back pain in many ways. Whenever there is a pinched nerve or nerve pressure, whether caused by a herniated disc or a muscle imbalance, inflammation also will be present as the body struggles to heal the injury. Overworked muscles often are inflamed, contributing to pain and delaying healing. Injuries cause inflammation, so if you've pulled, strained, or sprained a muscle or ligament, you'll have inflammation. And new studies are looking into the possibility that inflammation may damage nerves to the point that they signal chronic pain even when no injury is present.

In other words, both nerve-based back pain and tissue-based back pain (i.e., trigger points, muscle pain, and ligament and tendon pain) involve inflammation in the pain process.

What Does Diet Have to Do With It?

So why are we in inflammation overdrive, and what does diet have to do with it? In a word, everything. In fact, when asked why we're experiencing more inflammation these days, the really sharp doctors and scientists will typically point first to diet. Basically, we're eating too much of the foods that cause inflammation and too little of those that cool it.

Let's step back in time for a moment. Our ancestors, those prehistoric humans, were much less likely to have the inflammatory diseases of today. When we look for reasons why, we know, for one, that their diets were very different from ours.

First of all, they were hunters and gatherers, so they tended to eat lean meat, berries, roots, and other plants. This was a diet high in protein, fiber, and complex carbohydrates (foods that take a while to break down and are less likely to be stored as fat). In other words, it was a diet high in "good" fats (omega-3 fatty acids) and low in the "bad" fats that actually stimulate inflammation (omega-6 fatty acids found in shortening, margarine, refined grains, and trans fats). They ate no processed foods, like white flour, and no refined sugar. Finally, with their high intake of fruits and vegetables, they consumed a lot of antioxidants, which help the body fight inflammation. And, something that many people don't realize, the soil hundreds of years ago was much richer in nutrients than it is today and there weren't nearly the same levels of toxic chemicals in the water or soil.

Fast forward to today, when we have the exact opposite situation. Now that we've moved from the hunter-gatherer diet to one filled with refined grains, simple carbohydrates (foods that the body breaks down quickly and then stores as fat, such as baked goods, fruit juice, soda, and many sweetened cereals), fast food, processed foods such as white bread and ready-made meals, and an abundance of sweets, our systems are overwhelmed with inflammatory agents.

In general, we eat too many foods that contain the bad omega-6 fats and not enough of those that contain the good omega-3 fats. This creates an imbalance in the body, which encourages inflammation. Vegetable oils such as safflower, sunflower, corn, and soy contain more of those bad fats that encourage inflammation. Grains such as wheat also have been shown to create inflammation in the body. And while some "experts" will claim that "red meat" such as beef is bad for you, the fact is, it's only bad if the cow was fed refined grains instead of grass.

Then you have dairy...many people consume huge amounts of dairy, almost always from sick cows, which again have been fed refined grains and often given no room to roam like they would in the wild.

Massive amounts of sugar (in sweets, sodas, even everyday foods such as cereal, ketchup, and soups) also encourage inflammation through the release of certain hormones. Processed foods contain artificial colors and flavors as well as chemicals such as MSG and BHT that the body sees as invaders and tries to fight off, again increasing the rescue effort.

Meanwhile, we have fewer antioxidants to fight off these ill effects. We're using up the calories we consume every day on low-nutrient foods, thereby failing to give our bodies the fruits, vegetables, and other warrior-packed foods they need to heal. This puts more stress on the body and—you guessed it—causes more inflammation as the body struggles to right itself.

The Hidden Dangers of Excess Body Fat

A poor diet can cause you to gain weight, which can strain your back and exacerbate muscle imbalances. You probably already know that if you're overweight, it throws off your body's center of gravity. Let's say you have extra weight in your belly area. That weight draws your waist and hips forward. You can picture the pressure this creates on your back, curving your spine more than normal and overworking your discs.

Extra abdominal or lower body weight also can add strain to your joints and muscles. Basically, you may be carrying around an extra 20, 30, 40, or more pounds with you wherever you go. This extra weight overloads the joints and pulls muscles off balance as they struggle to adjust to the postural dysfunction.

But I'm going to tell you something else here that may surprise you. Body fat can cause you pain not only because it changes your body structure, but also because it helps contribute to internal inflammation! The cells that store excess energy as fat produce other cells that stimulate inflammation. As they swell up to store more fat, they produce more cells that activate the inflammation response. Excess body fat that surrounds organs such as the heart, liver, and stomach seem to have the biggest effect on inflammation. Scientists have found that organ fat is crawling with immune cells, keeping the inflammation going and damaging surrounding tissues.

To be clear, I'm talking about body fat, not dietary fat. For example, eating nuts, fish, or meats, which are full of healthy fats, is not bad unless of course you eat way too much (excess).

A Shortage of Your Body's Natural Anti-Inflammation Agents

In addition to diet, there is another reason inflammation can get out of control: a lack of natural anti-inflammatories.

Up until about age 27, the body produces an abundance of a special type of enzymes (called proteolytic enzymes) that "turn off" the inflammation when the repair work is done. But after that age, the production of these enzymes drops off dramatically. That's why once you hit that age, you start to "feel old." You don't recover as fast, your joints get stiff and achy, and a simple cut that used to heal in a few days can now take weeks.

These enzymes are natural anti-inflammatories. Unfortunately, as we get older, our bodies produce less of them. This is why older people seem to suffer more from inflammation-related problems of all types. They have less ability to turn off the inflammation process.

What does this mean for the body? Damage, damage, and more damage.

Here's Why Your Joints are Stiff, Tight, and Achy

We've discussed how inflammation can cause back pain if it's present around the spine, in the muscles of the back, or throughout the body, creating a general inflammation overdrive that reduces our ability to fight off everyday stress and strain. But there's one more thing that will make the connection between inflammation and back pain even clearer: Inflammation can be a sign that your body is producing excess fibrin.

Fibrin is a protein deposit that remains after an injury has healed.

Another term for it is scar tissue. It's deposited around the wound in the form of mesh, like a webbed foundation, creating a framework on which new tissue can grow. In a healthy body, it works to encourage healing, but in an unhealthy, inflamed body, it will accumulate too much, clumping together and creating excess scar tissue.

Imagine a large scab on the knuckle of your finger. While you have it, your finger will not bend as easily as usual and will not feel as flexible. The same thing happens if excess scar tissue forms on your tendons, ligaments, muscles, or other connective tissues. It limits your range of motion and makes moving more of a chore. It's as if a layer of chicken wire has been attached to various sections of your body, making it more difficult to bend, twist, and stretch. Excess fibrin can cause arthritis, back pain, fibromyalgia, and pain in any joint.

The situation worsens if the fibrin attaches itself to blood vessels. This restricts blood flow, making it harder for your body to get nutrient-rich blood to the areas that need healing. This is one of the reasons why older people take longer to heal than younger people—they carry more scar tissue in their bodies.

The Body's Solution

The body does have a solution for fibrin. Remember those enzymes I mentioned? In addition to regulating inflammation, they also break down fibrin so it can be whisked away with the rest of the waste. When we're younger, we have plenty of these enzymes to do their work, and our bodies, once they're healed, remain as flexible and springy as they were before.

As we grow older, however, the body doesn't produce as many of these enzymes—plus they're overworked trying to deal with all the inflammation inside us—so we have fewer enzymes to break down the fibrin. Thus, the scar tissue remains, where it can continue to cause stiffness and more inflammation.

Since these enzymes also help block pain-producing messengers (prostaglandins), having fewer enzymes means we're going to experience more of the pain our bodies signal. In other words, that operator in the spinal cord is going to send more and more pain messages through to the brain, rather than letting a few slide, as it might do when there are more enzymes around. The brain will be assaulted with pain message after pain message, and there's no button to silence the ring!

The Medical Doctor's Approach to Inflammation

Most doctors approach muscular inflammation, such as back pain, by prescribing prescription and over-the-counter anti-inflammatory drugs. The most popular in this category (known as NSAIDs—non-steroidal anti- inflammatory drugs) is ibuprofen.

The doctor's reasoning is that if the muscles in your body are "on fire" (i.e., inflamed), he'll hose them down with "cooling" anti-inflammatory drugs.

At first glance, this seems perfectly reasonable. Got a fire? Spray water on it to extinguish the blaze. But there are a few major drawbacks to this approach.

First, when your body is in a state of permanent inflammation, you can put out the "fire" with these drugs, but unless you cut off the source of the fuel, the inflammation will just come back.

Imagine a 500-gallon propane tank that is leaking propane—just enough to catch fire, but not enough to explode the tank. You could approach this situation by trying to hose down the fire. However, unless you stop the leak completely, the fire could be sparked again by something as simple as static cling.

The second limitation of anti-inflammatory drugs is that, since they were intended for short-term use, they can have serious side effects with prolonged use. Your liver, for instance—the organ that cleanses your blood of things that don't normally belong there (like these drugs)—can tolerate light use of these drugs once in a while, but as the warning labels tell you, it can't continue doing so for more than a few days at most.

Finally, the third limitation of using anti-inflammatories is that you're not doing anything to increase your body's natural anti-inflammatory agents—namely, certain foods and enzymes. Unlike the anti-inflammatory drugs, your body can easily handle long-term consumption of anti-inflammatory foods and proteolytic enzyme supplements.

In an upcoming section of this book on solutions for living a pain free life, I'll talk more about which foods actually calm inflammation and how to naturally supplement your anti-inflammatory proteolytic enzyme levels.

Meanwhile, in the next chapter, let's put everything we've learned together and see where you stand on the three areas of pain.

CHAPTER 9

HOW THE BODY, MIND, AND DIET INTERACT

Health is a state of complete harmony of the body, mind and spirit. When one is free from physical disabilities and mental distractions, the gates of the soul open.
B.K.S. Iyengar

As you read the preceding chapters, you may have been thinking: Does this apply to me? Is this my problem?

It's good to ask yourself this. After all, you're reading this book to find out what you can do to get rid of your back pain and live a healthier, more comfortable life.

At this point, however, I want to make something clear: You may not find a single, easy answer. Your pain cycle will likely involve more than one—or even all three—pain areas.

Most of us want things to be simple. It's easier for us. In other words, if you could determine that your pain is originating from the emotional burdens in your mind, then you'd have the solution: Create balance in your mind and emotions. That could include adopting stress-management techniques, visiting with a psychiatrist or psychologist, or simplifying your life with fewer demands and activities. Done. Check back pain off your list.

While solving back pain may sometimes be this simple, it's usually a bit more complicated.

Your body, mind, and diet aren't stand-alone islands. Everything interacts and weaves together. Imagine a plate of spaghetti. Some noodles are emotions, some are diet, some are the physical body, but they all intertwine, continuously acting on each other and feeding the effects back to you and your life.

This is why it's so difficult for doctors to properly diagnose back pain. For one, they simply don't take the time. The demands of their jobs—to say nothing of the demands of insurance companies—mean that they spend only a few minutes with you. It's near impossible to determine in 15 minutes all the different things that may be contributing to your back pain.

Second, most medical doctors aren't aware of how the mind, body, and diet can all affect your condition. Even if they are, they may not use that knowledge when treating your back pain. Instead, they're going to follow their training, which is to diagnose the physical source of the pain and address it with drugs, surgery, or a referral to a specialist.

Of course, you now know that this approach will only partially (if at all) address the problem. The three areas that contribute to pain— mind, body, and diet—all interact and influence each other. It's very important to carefully and objectively review all three areas in your life in order to increase your odds of living pain free.

An Example: Job Stress

Imagine a time when your career was exceptionally stressful and demanding. Maybe you were just promoted and trying to step up to the new position, or perhaps you were concerned about losing your job and were working extra hard to keep it.

In either of those situations, multiple factors might lead to back pain. Let's visualize the complete scenario.

Say your job involved some type of computer work, so you sat at a desk all day. You put in longer hours than usual, kept breaks short, and ate lunch without getting up. Your time in the sitting position increased—putting you at greater risk for muscle imbalances. Under normal circumstances, a light muscle imbalance can be kept in check by frequent standing and walking to stretch the legs, hips, and other muscles.

But if you went through several weeks of "crunch time," your habits may have subtly changed without you realizing it. You may have skipped some—or a lot—of those breaks away from your desk.

Let's also say that as part of your job you spent time on the phone. Maybe you were in sales, coordinating a project, or serving demanding clients. During "crunch time," you probably spent even more time on the phone than you normally would have. Maybe you typically used a headset, but it broke and you didn't have a chance to get it replaced. Since you were on a deadline, you used the regular handset and wedged it between your ear and neck. Knowing what you know now, you can see that the situation set you up for a bout with neck pain. The awkward position of the neck could very easily have pinched a nerve. And the lengthy period of time in the sitting position could screw up the natural tilt of your pelvis, pressuring nerves in the lower part of your spinal cord.

At the same time, all those hours of sitting caused the muscles in your rear end to suffer from insufficient blood circulation, which can contribute to the development of a trigger point. As if all this weren't enough, let's look at what could have been going on in your life from a mind and diet standpoint. The challenges at work most likely increased your stress load. If you're like most people, when you're stressed, your breathing becomes shallow. Deep breaths are great at bringing in more oxygen and helping you to relax, but if you're taking shallow breaths, you're missing out on this important benefit. The result is too much stress, too little relaxation, and too little oxygen, contributing to, or "activating," trigger points in the muscles.

So, now you have back pain caused (or made worse) by the emotional or stressful burdens in your mind. But wait, it gets worse.

In the midst of all this work and stress, it was probably difficult to eat well. Perhaps you drank more coffee in the morning to get going, increasing your caffeine levels. Maybe you skipped breakfast to get to work earlier. By lunchtime, you were starving, so you snacked on potato chips with their high levels of processed carbohydrates and unhealthful omega-6 fats.

By afternoon, you may have repeated the process of coffee (with lots of sugar), more potato chips, and maybe a cookie. Instead of drinking water like you used to, you stuck with coffee and caffeinated soda, thinking they would hydrate you just as well. Little did you realize that caffeine is a diuretic that forces water from your body, leaving you dehydrated.

So what were the consequences of all these changes?

All the junk food you ate also was pain- and inflammation-enhancing food. This increased the pain level in your body. Meanwhile, since you ate few healthful foods, you lacked the natural anti-inflammatories that would have increased your pain tolerance.

At the same time, as a result of the dehydration, there was too little water in your blood. This shifted the ratio of water to toxins, which had two impacts: The higher level of waste products in your blood stimulated more inflammation, and the toxins accumulated in major muscle areas, such as in your back, in the form of trigger points or knots—giving you back pain, caused by diet.

In this hypothetical example, I've given an extreme-case scenario to show how the body, mind, and diet can all independently cause back pain—and how all three areas combine to exacerbate the problem.

You can apply this general idea to any stressful period in your life, and soon you'll begin to see how all these areas interact and contribute to back pain.

Resolving Back Pain from Multiple Causes

When you have a situation like the previous example, or any other stressful situation, it helps to write down (or verbally record) what's going on. In our example, the overall lifestyle change was "crunch time at work." You may have experienced (or be currently experiencing) a death in the family, a divorce, an injury, or any number of other life changes. During these times, you'll want to record what you're feeling and note the major behavioral changes with respect to your physical habits (related to the body), the stress and emotional concerns burdening your mind, and the diet you adopt.

When you write down these behaviors, you can see how they are interconnected. In the example we used, you could opt to treat any one of the three areas—body, mind, or diet—to begin with. But frankly, when you're able to see the big picture, you'll realize that it's the job situation (or other life event) that's causing all the damaging changes.

If changing the career situation is impossible in the short run, you may opt for treating the problems in your body, mind, and diet. However, if you can somehow change or improve the job situation (or any other stressful situation in your life), the issues in your body, mind, and diet may either disappear entirely (especially if you didn't suffer from back pain previously), or at least cause you less back pain, which could make it a lot easier to use the specific treatment approaches recommended later for the body, mind, and/or diet.

Solutions for a Pain Free Life

In the next section, we'll cover proven solutions available for a pain free life. I'll recommend major treatment approaches for the body, mind, and diet; explain when each should be used; and tell you why each works to solve specific back pain conditions. You'll find all the right "ingredients" or components to help solve your particular situation.

In the last section of the book, I'll present several seven-day action plans to solve common types of back pain conditions. These include lower back pain, upper back pain, sciatic pain, and many others. These action plans are like pain relief "recipes"—a slightly different one for each particular type of pain. Each one uses the "ingredients" in a specific order to best address the causes of the problem.

For now, let's look at how each of the major treatment approaches works—giving you an understanding of the role of each potential "ingredient."

PART II:

SOLUTIONS FOR A PAIN FREE LIFE

CHAPTER 10

WHY MOST BACK PAIN TREATMENTS FAIL

*The...patient should be made to understand that he
or she must take charge of his own life. Don't take your
body to the doctor as if he were a repair shop.*
Quentin Regestein

When you have back pain, a variety of health care specialists stand ready to serve you. Medical doctors, orthopedic surgeons, chiropractors, physical therapists, acupuncturists, and massage therapists. For some back pain sufferers, these professionals may prove helpful, but for a surprisingly high number of others, specialists only ease pain—or maybe eliminate it temporarily—*without solving the underlying causes of that pain.*

Some people, no matter what specialist they go to, or even if they use a combination of two or more, have recurring pain. In the meantime they may suffer unnecessarily, through multiple surgeries, injections, and prescription drug use (which can increase stress on the body), to say nothing of the drain on a bank account and the strain placed on the spirit.

So, why do people keep going to these professionals if they're not helping? Probably because the treatments help *a little.* They can ease pain, loosen tight muscles, and even right a postural dysfunction—for a short time.

Let's review the most common professionals back pain sufferers turn to for help—and the limitations of each of their approaches.

Professional #1: The Medical Doctor

Medical doctors are great at treating trauma and emergencies. If you are in a serious car accident, medical doctors are likely going to be your best chance for survival. However, the same professionals who have impressive track records for treating trauma have comparatively poor success rates at resolving everyday aches and pains.

In a trauma, the cause of the problem is very obvious. If you're in a car accident and end up with a broken leg, it's clear what caused the problem. It's clear what's "broken" with your body. And it's equally clear to doctors what they need to do to fix you.

But with everyday aches and pains, it's not always so easy to determine the cause. Often, there are multiple contributing factors. But medical doctors—who are trained to look for "the problem"—by their very nature zoom in and focus on the back. Consequently, they'll ask you what you were doing before you "threw out" your back.

Once you answer that question, the doctor thinks he's found the problem. He tells you to be more careful next time (i.e., don't bend from the waist, which is horrible advice by the way), drugs you up until the pain goes away, and believes the problem has been solved.

Medical doctors aren't trained to examine the three areas of body, mind, and diet. Even if they were, they wouldn't have the time. A thorough examination of every aspect of your life overall—and your body, mind, and diet, specifically—takes much longer than the typical 8-to-15-minute doctor visit.

When I assess a back pain sufferer, it always takes me one to two hours (or longer) to do a thorough job. I'm looking at posture; examining muscle strength of various muscle pairs; testing range of motion and flexibility; and observing how a person walks, stands, leans over, tilts, sits, and more. I'm trying to understand the overall context of what's going on in the person's life. Is he going through a job change? Did he just get married or divorced? Did he just move?

I'm also looking to understand his dietary habits—what does he eat or drink, how often, and why? How does his diet fit into his overall life? How is everything connected?

The Typical Doctor Visit for Back Pain

If you have back pain, most likely the doctor is going to zoom in on the back as the problem. He's not going to look at your posture, your feet, your knees, or your hips. He probably won't ask about your diet or the stress in your life. Most likely, he won't take a blood test to examine the levels of nutrients in your system, hormone imbalances, or the like. He doesn't have time or he doesn't even know to look in these places. If the problem is in your back, he'll look at your back, make an assessment, maybe send you for X-rays, and come up with a solution. And that solution will, the majority of the time, be a drug or a referral to a specialist. It's what he's been trained to do.

This tunnel vision means that the doctor figures your problem is pain, inflammation, or nerve pressure or damage—or some combination of these—and that he, therefore, must fix these problems. Prescribing anti-inflammatory drugs is often the first thing he'll do. The inflammation must be controlled. He's right about that—we want to reduce the inflammation—but the problem is that drug-based anti-inflammatories are often hard on the body. Although they may mask the problem temporarily by providing pain relief, they don't offer a long-term solution.

Popular recommendations typically come in the form of over-the-counter or prescription non-steroidal anti-inflammatory drugs, or NSAIDs. Most are familiar with many of these drug options already, like ibuprofen, naproxen, or celecoxib. However, since they don't solve the underlying problem (which could be in the mind, body, and/or diet), the patient ends up having to use them again and again.

Prolonged use of NSAIDs increases the probability of stomach ulcers and intestinal bleeding. They're also hard on the kidneys and liver. For people who are experiencing chronic pain and popping pills on a regular basis, the risks can become serious, indeed.

Your medical doctor also may prescribe muscle relaxers. If you're suffering from a muscle imbalance, muscle relaxers will grant you temporary relief. If muscle tightness has you "locked up" in a certain position (if you've experienced a muscle spasm), these drugs can relieve the rigidity and help you get moving again. If your muscles are putting pressure on a nerve (as in sciatica), have caused a herniated disc, or have become so chronically tight that you're suffering from fibromyalgia, you're only going to gain temporary relief with these pills.

But again, the doctor is addressing only the pain—not the reason for the pain. So, most likely, as soon as you stop taking the prescription drug, that pain is going to come back. Also, it's important to point out that there are safer, natural alternatives, such as valerian, white willow bark, chamomile, and magnesium, as well as homeopathics, such as arnica and kali carb, just to name a few.

Professional #2: The Orthopedic Specialist

All right, let's say the doctor's prescriptions helped for a while, but the pain returned. In most cases, he'll now recommend you to a specialist, often an orthopedic specialist. This is a medical professional who specializes in the muscles, ligaments, bones, tendons, joints, and nerves—all the parts of the body responsible for allowing us to move.

The orthopedic specialist (surgeon) is going to focus on the structural issues of your body—looking for major trauma and injury. If you have a herniated disc, she's going to zoom in on how to "repair that disc." She may say something like, "Your MRI shows bulging and/or herniated discs at L4-L5, L5-S1" (referring to the specific vertebrae affected).

When you hear a verbal version of this report, it seems so clinical and certain. A particular vertebra or disc appears to be in an abnormal position—which may be factually true. But what's not necessarily true is that the vertebra that's in the abnormal position, or the bulging disc, is actually pressing the nerve that's been causing you pain. That's just an educated guess.

The surgeon's next response is to tell you, "I'd like to go in and clean it up." She's going to either remove a piece of the disc with scissors and knives or burn it with a laser. The idea is that once that "offending" piece of the disc is gone, it will no longer put pressure on the nerve, thereby relieving your pain. Again, this assumes that a specific disc is actually pressing on a nerve and that that specific nerve is the one causing your pain.

Here's the problem: That bulging disc may not even be the culprit. In fact, in a study published in *The New England Journal of Medicine*, researchers found that 28 percent of the MRIs they analyzed with disc herniations belonged to people who had reported never having back pain!

Discs often erode as we get older, but whether or not they bother us is dependent upon the person. In addition, many studies show that when left alone, most herniated discs will heal on their own, often in just months. With time, they often are absorbed back into the spine or, if torn, they heal, just like a cut on your skin does.

While the presurgical experience seems like a very scientific one, at some point in the process, it deviates from factual science and becomes educated guessing based on factual science.

What almost never happens is the surgeon probing into the reasons why you have pain or a disc herniation. They don't ask, "What caused the disc to move into that abnormal position in the first place?"

Without this probing—if muscle imbalances caused the herniated disc in the first place, for instance—that underlying problem hasn't been solved. Even with surgery, the muscle imbalances within your body have not been rebalanced. Over time, your surgically repaired discs will face the same pressures and, likely, end up bulging all over again.

From a surgeon's perspective, the solution will be simple: Perform the surgery to remove the offending disc...again. That's one of the many reasons why some people go through surgery after surgery. In many cases, the surgeon isn't cutting out the problem, just the symptom—leaving the problem to cause more pain in the future.

If your pain persists and you don't want surgery, many orthopedic surgeons will recommend cortisone shots. Cortisone injections, epidurals, steroid injections, and epidural steroid injections are all essentially the same thing. The goal is to inject a chemical into the inflamed area and try to control the inflammation, delivering relief in the short term.

Some people feel better by the time they get home, or perhaps the next morning. However, others don't feel better at all. It's about a 50/50 chance. Because the effects last only a few weeks, you may have to go back for two, three, maybe more shots, until you reach the limit. And there is a limit, because too much cortisone in the tissues can result in permanent damage, weakening tendons or causing deterioration in the cartilage of the joint.

How does this happen? Cortisone shots can cause harm in two ways. First, because cortisone is a type of steroid that inhibits inflammation, it also halts healing. Injecting an injured area may relieve pain, but at the same time, it sends the body's repair service home, leaving the area defenseless and weak. The patient, believing he's cured, goes back to working the joint, muscle, or tendon, not realizing he could be doing further damage.

Second, cortisone is a catabolic steroid, which tends to break down and destroy connective tissues. Actual cell death is seen near the injection site. So most doctors set the limit at two to three shots (although I have one client who received nine!). Regardless of the outcome, if the underlying cause wasn't addressed, the pain will return.

Of course, not all orthopedic specialists recommend surgery right off the bat. It depends on your condition and on the specialist. Many will suggest rest, physical therapy, specially constructed back supports and braces, or safety belts. Again, these can be helpful in temporarily alleviating pain, but they don't address the range of underlying problems that may be causing the pain.

Professional #3: The Chiropractor

Let's say you bypassed the shots and surgical options and went, instead, to a local chiropractor. You knew he wasn't going to put you under the knife, so you figured it was a safer choice.

Chiropractors deal with the spine and surrounding tissues and how they can affect the rest of the body through the nervous system. If something is wrong, chiropractors believe your spine is out of alignment, causing interruption to the signals coming from your brain. For nerve-based back pain, this can be true—in some cases. However, if the pressured nerve is located in an area other than the spine, say, the sciatic nerve as it passed by the piriformis muscle, then the vertebrae in the back aren't necessarily to blame.

A chiropractor believes that through manipulation of the spine itself and the surrounding soft tissues he can bring the body back into alignment, which will then help the nerve signals and impulses flow as they should, resulting in less pain. While this approach can work, for many people it often fails because it addresses only some of the causes.

The biggest drawback of using a chiropractor is the duration of the pain relief. If you have nerve-based back pain and a chiropractor realigns your spine correctly, you may feel pain relief—until the muscle imbalances that caused your spine to become misaligned in the first place undoes the chiropractor's adjustments. For nerve-based back pain, the most common reason for spinal misalignments is muscle imbalances. These imbalances are not addressed completely through the spinal manipulations performed by chiropractors.

If you're suffering from an intensely painful episode of nerve-based back pain, a spinal adjustment will typically provide relief for 12 to 48 hours. At that point, the muscle imbalances will put unequal pressure on various parts of your spine, causing the vertebrae to be pulled out of alignment once again.

The chiropractor's solution for such a severe case is to have you come in for an adjustment every 48 hours—typically three times a week—until the pain goes away permanently. Typically, this involves two to four months of treatment, or until your insurance runs out.

If this seems like an incomplete solution to you, I'd agree.

But I do think good chiropractic care *combined with Muscle Balance Therapy* is a very effective approach to treating back pain. Chiropractic treatments get your spine into alignment, and Muscle Balance Therapy keeps it there. When the two are paired together, the number of chiropractic treatments needed is reduced dramatically and the chance of another back pain episode drops drastically.

However, without Muscle Balance Therapy, chiropractic care for nerve-based back pain is just a very expensive way to buy 24 to 48 hours of relief.

Also, keep in mind that if your back pain originates in the muscles—as trigger points—then chiropractic manipulation is practically useless. The only exception is if the trigger point is so severe that it causes a muscle imbalance and nerve-based back pain. In these "double whammy" situations in which you're suffering from both types of back pain, chiropractic care paired with Muscle Balance Therapy could solve half the problem.

Unfortunately, there are few chiropractors who are even aware of the muscle balance approach, so if you're going to work with a chiropractor, understand that you'll likely need to do additional treatments, such as Muscle Balance Therapy and trigger point therapy, to get lasting relief.

Professional #4: The Physical Therapist

Any of the professionals we've talked about so far could, at any time, recommend you to a physical therapist (PT). There are several types of PTs, including geriatric and neurological, but typically someone with spinal problems will go to an orthopedic PT (or neurological PT, for an actual spinal cord injury).

Orthopedic PTs deal with disorders and injuries in the muscles, tendons, ligaments, joints, and bones. Most of their work is done in an outpatient clinical setting, where they help people recover and regain movement after surgery. They are trained to deal with patients recovering from postoperative procedures, such as sports injuries, amputations, fractures, sprains, strains, and neck and back pain.

The idea behind most physical therapy is that you've had an injury (and/or an operation) and the muscle, tendon, or joint is now weak or limited in range of motion, so you need to build it back up to normal. It's very similar in the case of back pain, even if you haven't had surgery. The PT's job will be to get you moving and get you strong. As with the chiropractic method, whatever exercises or treatments the PT prescribes will be based on your pain symptoms, not the underlying cause of those symptoms.

Let's say you have that herniated disc again. The PT is going to recommend the same exercises to you that she would to anyone else who has a herniated disc. Unfortunately, since these exercises are not tailored to your particular dysfunctions or muscle imbalances, they have a low success rate. The exercises may help you in other ways, perhaps stretching or strengthening some muscles, but if those muscles are not the ones you need stretched or strengthened, the exercises could actually make your condition worse.

PTs also use heat, which can loosen up your muscles, but then again, so can a hot tub or far infrared heat. Additional tools include ice, which can help control inflammation in the early stages of injury; ultrasound, which helps increase blood flow, stimulate healing, break up scar tissue, and control inflammation (but which can only be used limited times and with limited effects); and electrical stimulation, which can help stimulate and strengthen very weak muscles. All these tools may help ease pain for a short time and might even relax some muscles that are in spasm, but that's as far as they'll go.

What often happens with modern physical therapy is similar to what happens in today's doctor offices—most practitioners don't take enough time to do a thorough evaluation. In addition, since the PT relies on the doctor to refer patients, she will rarely question or change the prescription the doctor gave you. She'll read the doctor's diagnosis as "back pain" and proceed to treat the symptoms—without investigating the cause of that pain. You may go through a series of exercises, but months or years later, you still may be in pain.

The one-size-fits-all bias of PTs limits their usefulness. Just because two people feel back pain in their upper back doesn't mean they both have the same underlying problem. For example, one person could have tissue-based back pain due to poor circulation caused by dietary imbalances and mental stress. The other could have severe muscle imbalances. To really solve these two problems, they must be approached differently—even though both people feel pain in the same part of the body.

This lack of a personalized approach—based on the specific conditions within your body, diet, and mind—largely explains the hit-or-miss track record that PTs have with resolving back pain, or any other ailment for that matter.

Professional #5: The Acupuncturist

Many people get fed up with popping pills all the time, so they look for an alternative method of pain relief. Acupuncture can be one of those alternatives. An ancient Chinese practice, acupuncture involves inserting hair-thin, sterile needles into specific body parts to stimulate healing and pain relief. It also uses heat, Chinese massage, exercise, diet, herbs, and a practice called "cupping," in which a partial vacuum is created in cups placed on the skin either by means of heat or suction.

Acupuncture operates on the premise that we each contain vital energy flowing through our bodies via invisible channels called "meridians." An imbalance in that flow is believed to precede pain and dysfunction.

Acupuncturists insert needles along these meridian lines to restore the balance of energy flow. It's believed to work by releasing feel-good endorphins, stimulating circulation, and influencing the nerve impulses and electrical currents of the body. The practice of cupping is believed to relieve energy stagnation, encourage blood flow, and release toxins.

Acupuncture is much more likely to be helpful to people who suffer from tissue-based back pain (e.g., trigger points), where the pain is triggered by poor circulation and the resulting buildup of toxins. The improved circulation that results from acupuncture is a good match for this type of back pain.

However, acupuncture has two important limitations. First, for back pain caused by trigger points, it can help resolve the toxin buildup in the trigger point area, but it doesn't address why the buildup occurred in the first place. For example, if you consume a diet that encourages toxin buildup or suffer mental stress that contributes to poor blood circulation, acupuncture won't address these underlying causes. It only will work as a short-term pain-reduction treatment that will have to be repeated frequently.

Second, acupuncture's impact on nerve-based back pain is much more limited. Treatments can improve the body's ability to tolerate a higher level of pain, which can be beneficial temporarily, but it isn't a great solution for physically moving vertebrae and muscles away from irritated nerves.

While acupuncture has value as a secondary form of back pain relief, since it doesn't address all the underlying causes, it's not a great standalone or primary back pain relief solution.

Professional #6: The Massage Therapist

Many different forms of massage therapy exist, with varying degrees of usefulness for back pain sufferers.

First, you have the general "relaxation," or "Swedish," style of massage, which, while it can't address the underlying causes of your pain, can be very helpful at reducing stress and relaxing muscles.

Then you have "deep tissue," or "sports," massage, which can be effective at reducing or eliminating back pain when combined with Muscle Balance Therapy and other treatments. By itself, however, it will rarely be enough to provide lasting relief. It also tends to produce quite a bit of discomfort both during the massage and afterward, so many patients tend to give up on it rather quickly. And if the therapist is not well-trained or familiar with your body and situation, deep tissue massage may end up aggravating things as opposed to relaxing them. I personally only get relaxation massages because I always find that I feel worse after a deep tissue massage, in part because it often activates trigger points that were dormant.

So Which Treatment Approaches Work?

We can begin to see the many limitations of the more popular types of back pain treatments. If you've tried some of these approaches with unsatisfactory results, I hope these explanations help you to better understand why.

While the more common forms of back pain treatment have their shortcomings, it doesn't mean that all available treatments don't work. In fact, many treatments and combinations of treatments work quite well—especially when applied to the right situation. This is the focus of the next chapter.

CHAPTER 11

THE SOLUTION FOR A PAIN FREE LIFE

The part can never be well unless the whole is well.
Plato

The solution for a pain free life is based on two essential rules. First, you must focus on the cause of the pain, not just the symptoms. Second, you must do some investigating to determine the cause, realizing it will very likely consist of more than one element in your life. When these two rules are broken, you get recurring back pain.

Long-term relief comes from concentrating on the source of the pain. However, if you're experiencing debilitating pain right now that prevents you from adopting the recommended strategies coming up, I'll give you a few temporary pain relief techniques that can get you feeling well enough to implement the more permanent solutions.

Rule #1: Focus on the Cause, Not Just the Symptom

To enjoy a pain free life, you have to see pain/symptom management for what it really is—temporary. When fixing major catastrophic traumas, medical doctors are quite successful. For example, if you break a bone and it's not able to heal properly on its own, the surgeons can use screws to get the pieces of bone back in place so they can heal.

But back pain isn't like a broken bone and, in most cases, it isn't a trauma, either. The causes aren't so obvious, the usefulness of medical testing is less conclusive, and the medical treatment track record is mediocre at best (as you likely know firsthand).

Consequently, most treatment approaches focus primarily on short-term pain relief—rather than delving into the underlying causes of the pain. For example, doctors diagnose the problem as a herniated disc, sciatica, muscle strain, etc., and prescribe a solution. Rarely are these questions asked: "What caused the sciatic nerve to flare up in the first place?" or "What caused the disc to rupture anyway?" In the case of back pain, such questions absolutely must be asked—and answered—if you are to live a pain free life.

Unfortunately, doctors rarely entertain these questions—which is a major reason why so many people suffer from recurring back pain. If you want to eliminate your back pain once and for all, you have to ask—and answer—the question of the cause(s).

Rule #2: Go "Upstream" to Find the Original Cause of Your Pain

To find the underlying cause of your back pain, you have to start with the symptom—pain—and work your way "upstream." When you do, you'll discover that all *back pain starts from issues with excesses, deficiencies, and stagnations in your mind, body, and diet.* A disruption in the delicate balance of these things is the underlying cause of all back pain. When you have too much of something in your life, too little of something, or blood circulation or qi (energy flow) that's too slow, you disrupt your body's ability to exist pain free.

The key is to define precisely what you have too much of, *what* you have too little of, and what is causing circulation that's too slow. When you're able to isolate these imbalances, you've discovered the secret to getting rid of your pain permanently. Also, it's important to note that this process works for all health ailments, not just back pain.

This process of isolating the underlying problem does take

some investigation. It's the most challenging part of getting better. Once you've actually figured it out, in most cases, it's quite easy to solve—with the majority of people experiencing significant or complete pain relief within seven days or less. However, the investigative part can sometimes take longer, especially if your back pain comes from several layers of causes.

In the chapters remaining in this section of the book, we'll cover the major treatment approaches that work. I'll explain under what conditions the approaches are useful, what limitations they have, and why they work. In the last section of the book (on action plans), I'll recommend specific approaches—which treatments to use and in which order, based on your particular situation.

Beware of the "No More Pain" Temptation

Many back pain sufferers are tempted to stop the process of solving their back pain problems the second the pain stops. This is a powerful temptation! However, just because the pain stops doesn't mean the problem is gone.

I've worked with many back pain sufferers over the years, and I've found that they fall into two categories: the "thoroughs" and the "just enoughs." The "thoroughs" figure out what's causing their pain and solve it once and for all. The "just enough" also figure it out, but then do just enough to take the edge off. But—and this is the critical difference—these people are now so attuned to what's causing the problem, they can detect the warning signs before a full-blown backache happens. When they do get a warning, they use the treatment approaches you're about to learn in the next few chapters to once again take the edge off.

In an ideal world, it would be my hope that everyone would focus on getting rid of his or her pain once and for all. It does take a little more time to do, but it's so worth it.

However, I'm also realistic. People have busy lives. For some, just being able to control back pain like a thermostat—knowing precisely when it's getting worse and how to dial back the factors that lead to severe pain—is good enough.

I point out these two approaches so that you can make a realistic and informed choice for yourself.

Short-Term Pain Relief

A number of back-pain sufferers I work with tell me they're in way too much pain to take the steps needed for long-term relief. While they're looking forward to solving their back pain problem once and for all, they can barely move right now.

While the remaining chapters in this section discuss various types of long-term solutions, let me now address the topic of short-term pain relief. Sometimes it's necessary—so long as it doesn't become an excuse to avoid a long-term solution.

For most people, short-term pain relief involves taking some type of anti-inflammatory medication like ibuprofen. These medications were originally designed to be used only once in a while, but many people now rely on them on a daily basis. Considering the dangers— heavy use increases the probability of stomach ulcers and intestinal bleeding and also places enormous stress on the liver and kidneys—I tell people to avoid them because there are much safer and effective alternatives. Personally, I haven't taken an over-the-counter or prescription pain reliever in well over a decade! Pain is a sign that something is wrong in the body, so the first task is to find out exactly what the problem is and to set about fixing it. To handle the pain in the meantime, there are numerous things you can do. Here are just a few proven methods.

One of the most powerful, all-natural pain relievers is called proteolytic enzyme therapy, and it's been used in numerous countries since the 1960s. Proteolytic enzymes occur naturally in your body and are responsible for a number of functions. Overall, they help drive various reactions, including digestion, immune response, and toxic cleansing. If your body were a corporation, these enzymes would be "middle management"—heavily involved in all the everyday tasks that make your body work.

These are the same enzymes I mentioned in earlier chapters. They are the ones that tell the immune system when to shut down inflammation—acting as the body's natural anti-inflammatories, so to speak. They also help "clean up" excess scar tissue (fibrin) that occurs when your body repairs damaged tissues, essentially breaking it down so it can be carried away with the rest of the body's waste.

According to numerous studies, these enzymes help reduce inflammation, promote healing, and alleviate arthritis. Sounds similar to your current anti-inflammatory drug, right? Except these enzymes occur naturally in your body and don't have the side effects that medications can have. Since they also help break down stiffening scar tissue, they can help improve flexibility and mobility—a benefit you won't find with over-the-counter drugs.

Your body produces these enzymes naturally—especially if you're still fairly young, say, in your 20s. However, as you get into your 40s, 50s, 60s, or older, your body produces less and less of them. If you're in the latter category, you'll be happy to know that enzyme supplements exist that can add to your body's own natural, but diminishing, supply.

Anti-Inflammation Enzyme Supplements

Obviously, not all enzyme supplements are alike, so here are a few guidelines. First, you want to find a combination of enzymes and herbs specifically created to reduce inflammation and pain.

Your best bet is not one, but a blend of enzymes, combined with natural extracts that have a demonstrated ability to reduce inflammation, ease pain and swelling, and increase joint mobility and flexibility without harsh side effects. You don't want a standard "digestive" enzyme formula.

Second, you want to check how much of each of the ingredients is in a serving. Some supplements list them on the ingredient list so you know they're in there, but either they don't tell you how much is present or they have used such small amounts that they're not going to do you any good.

Next, you want to look at the "fillers" in the product. Those are the "other ingredients" listed below the supplement facts. Many manufacturers use them to help the ingredients "stick together," making the pill easier to package and ship, while others use them to fill their capsules or tablets and minimize their costs by reducing the amount of active ingredients used. They may add animal derivatives, preservatives, or artificial substances like titanium dioxide, magnesium stearate, and the like. Products with minimal fillers are best—even better would be if any extra ingredients are only natural ones.

Finally, you want to look at how the supplement is delivered. Hard tablets typically don't absorb as well as capsules, gel tabs, liquids and creams.

Finding a proteolytic enzyme product that is effective at relieving pain and promoting mobility isn't easy. Some seem to have the right ingredients but don't have enough of these ingredients in a daily dosage to do any good. Others have high quantities of some helpful ingredients but none of the others that work in concert for a better overall effect. Some don't even list the amounts of the ingredients, claiming a "proprietary blend."

After years of looking and not being satisfied with any of the formulations available, I finally gave up and decided to work with a major nutrition laboratory to create the formulation that my research showed to be most effective. It combined the best parts of the various supplements available, without their shortcomings. Plus, my team has spent several years testing and refining the formula to continue to improve its effectiveness.

The result is an all-natural formula called Heal-n-Soothe®, and you can learn more about it at **www.healnsoothe.com**.

Pain Relief Creams

In addition to a proteolytic enzyme supplement, you may want to consider a rub-on cream, one that you can apply directly on the area of pain.

You may already have something like this. Maybe it has a warming effect, giving you slight relief from muscle tension, but it also may irritate your skin, work for only a short time, smell terrible, or lack the power to really do any good. Fortunately, there are creams out there that are much more effective.

The nice thing about a quality cream is that it's *fast*—it can deliver almost immediate relief. So while you're waiting for the proteolytic enzyme supplement to be digested and go to work in your body, the right cream can help you start feeling better right away. You can apply it directly to the area of your body that hurts and get the muscles and joints moving again if they're stiff or locked up.

You also can use creams on a daily basis if you need to, without worrying about unhealthy side effects (provided the cream you are using is not full of toxic chemicals, which many are so read the label!). If you're having trouble sleeping because of pain, a good rub-on cream can provide the ease that you need to drift off comfortably. It's also the perfect take-along tool for pain that strikes while you're traveling, working, or out doing some other activity.

When looking for a quality product, I'd encourage you to watch for three things.

First, the cream should be made with natural ingredients. There are many botanical and organic substances that battle inflammation and pain. Some creams take advantage of them. Find one that blends them together in a way that works. Even better, find one that has scientific studies behind it.

Second, look for a product that does more than just create heat. Many of the creams on the market do only that, conveying the idea that if you feel heat, it must be working. Unfortunately, this isn't necessarily the case.

While heat can help loosen stiff muscles, if that's all the product does, it won't help you much. A quality cream will go beyond that. The formula should provide powerful antioxidants that not only neutralize harmful cells at the injury point, but also help reduce inflammation. The right ingredients will absorb into the skin and into the muscle tissue to go to work on the injured area, relieving pain through a number of approaches.

Finally, the product should do something to alleviate stiffness. I mentioned that heat can do this, but other ingredients have proven to be more effective at penetrating the source of the problem, relaxing tight muscle fibers, and allowing for better movement.

The only pain cream I recommend—which has been proven in clinical studies—can be found at **www.rubonrelief.com**.

Far Infrared Heat

Now, I know that when you're feeling pain, you may reach for a heating pad. It's a natural response, as we all know heat can soothe and relax tight and painful muscles. But seriously, have you ever experienced true relief with your regular heating pad? I mean, it warms the area for a while, which can make you feel a little better, but typically, the results don't last. That's because a heating pad doesn't penetrate very deeply. It warms the skin, but that's about as far as it goes, and what you need is heat that reaches deep into your muscles.

Unfortunately, regular heat won't do that, but there is a type of heat that will. Know that delicious, bone deep warmth you feel from the sun on a perfect summer day? That feeling comes from the sun's infrared rays. These are different types of waves than the ultraviolet ones that can contribute to sunburn. Infrared rays don't harm your skin and they make your muscles feel great. You can't see them, because they have a longer wavelength than visible light, but you can feel them.

Infrared light that is farthest from visible light is called "far infrared," and it has been used to promote healing for years. For example, a study of patients with chronic fatigue syndrome found considerable relief from symptoms with daily infrared treatment. Plus, numerous other studies have found it to help everything from effective fat burning to killing cancer cells.

The reason far infrared heat is so effective at soothing pain, relaxing muscles, improving circulation, and reducing fatigue is its ability to *penetrate*. Just like those invisible sunrays that go deep into your body, far infrared heat has been shown in scientific studies to actually sink 2 to 3 inches into muscles and ligaments. As it goes, it transfers light energy into heat energy, expanding blood vessels, improving circulation, and encouraging the healing process. And if you've ever lain out in the sun after a cool swim, you know how good it feels!

There are more benefits to this type of heat. As blood circulation improves, toxins break down and flush out of the body. Things like uric acid, sodium, metals, and fat-soluble toxins are all moved out of muscles and tissues, releasing the body's own strength and healing abilities. Blood pressure comes down, muscle cramps relax, oxygen transport increases, fatigue melts away, and more. And because the heat goes so deep into the tissues, the effects last for up to six hours, depending on how long you soak in the heat.

So how do you take advantage of this deep-penetrating pain reliever? There are several far infrared devices out there, from a small pad to four-person saunas. Regular (non-infrared) heating pads use high-temperature heat to attempt to deliver heat deep into your muscles, but those near-burning temperatures cause too much pain for most people. In comparison, far infrared heating pads use moderate-temperature heat at a particular wavelength (the far infrared wave-length) that penetrates deeply into your muscles naturally.

Learn more about far infrared heating pads
and how they can help relieve your back pain at
www.losethebackpain.com/heat

Stress Reduction

As soon as you experience pain, you'll probably also experience some level of stress. That stress could be caused by fear or worry—*What's wrong with me?* Sometimes receiving a diagnosis and knowing what's wrong creates even more stress. Regardless of the reason, any stress can manifest itself physically, causing muscle tension and tightness that only serves to exaggerate pain.

Becoming informed about your condition, its causes, and ways you can treat it will help to reduce or alleviate your fears and worries, thus reducing stress. Ultimately, the cycle of pain causing stress and stress causing more pain will stop, and as a result, you'll be able to notice relief in the level of pain you're experiencing.

Get Out of Bed

After surgery, patients are now encouraged to get out of bed, usually the same day or within 24 hours. It's proven that getting out of bed and returning to some level of activity as quickly as possible promotes faster healing. This is also true for back pain sufferers. Limit the amount of time spent lying down by getting up as consistently and continuously as possible. It might be for short durations at first, but you should notice that you're steadily able to increase the amount of time spent on your feet. This is a good activity which promotes healing, reduces pain, keeps your muscles active, and enhances a positive attitude.

Breathing Techniques

It can be beneficial to perform relaxation exercises. Slow, deep breathing is one such exercise that is very calming and puts the body and the mind in a state of deep relaxation. In this state, the muscles loosen and tension decreases, which lessens any pain you're experiencing. Another plus: it clears the mind, which naturally reduces stress.

Alice Burmeister, author of *The Touch of Healing*, offers thousands of different breathing techniques in her book. Breathing is a calming exercise that benefits the body in multiple ways, one of which is distributing oxygen throughout the blood. Oxygen can help reduce pain. Incorporate a breathing technique that works for you into your short-term pain management program. Breathe deeply, consciously and intentionally, inhaling and exhaling fully as you focus on each breath. Do this as often as you can every day, for several minutes or an hour. You'll notice that this type of breathing brings immediate relaxation, which also helps to alleviate tension, stress, and pain.

Sound Nutrition

There are foods that are healthy and foods that are unhealthy. Of course, it makes sense to eat as healthy as possible, but it's also very important to understand the role nutrition plays in our overall health. It's also true that some foods provide more than sustenance and nutrition—for example, fish oils can help reduce pain and inflammation. Look for foods that are fresh and natural and those that are high in vitamins and minerals. Steer away from foods with high fat or sugar content, those with empty calories, and processed foods that include a lot of additives, as well as any food that has little or no nutritional value.

Drinking water is also a must. Go for the eight glasses a day rule, or you can determine how much water your body needs by this formula: One-half an ounce for every pound of body weight. So, a person who weighs 100 pounds should drink 50 ounces of water a day. This will help flush toxins from the muscles and body and regenerate the fluids in your muscles, discs and joints.

To ensure you're getting the proper nutrition, take supplements or multi-vitamins on a daily basis. Some of these supplements, like systemic enzymes, can reduce pain and inflammation.

Supporting Devices

There are many support devices for back and neck pain. These can range from contoured pillows, mattresses, massaging seats or chairs, braces, etc. If a supporting device helps you in any way, consider using it. It might be something as simple as putting an extra pillow under your knees at night to redistribute your body weight when you're sleeping. By reducing the pain at any level, a device can lower any irritation in your day or night, which will help you rest and heal.

Ice and Heat

During the first 48 to 72 hours, ice should be applied to minimize inflammation. After that period, heat can be applied. Massaging the afflicted area with ice is a good way to use massage therapy in conjunction with ice, and it produces even more effective results.

When applying heat, you can use a heating pad or a hot pack, or the far infrared heat therapy previously discussed. Hot showers are another good way to apply heat to aches and pains. Think about how good it feels to stand under a hot shower, letting the water soothe and loosen your achy muscles. It helps circulate the blood and brings temporary pain relief.

Healing Arts

The healing arts include massage, acupuncture, Qigong, Aromatherapy, Bowen Therapy, Cranio-Sacral Therapy and other energy healing techniques. You probably won't expect one of these techniques to provide total healing and ease all of your pain, but in conjunction with other techniques and pain relief methods, they can help get you to the next level in your healing process.

Set Specific Pain Relief Goals

It's vital that you have the mindset that you can and will improve. Therefore, setting daily, weekly, monthly, and even yearly health-related goals are also recommended. Goals give you something to work toward and reinforce the attitude that progress is being made. In addition, as you achieve each goal, you're reminded that what you're doing is working, that you're improving and feeling better than you did yesterday, last month, or last year.

Goals work because they confirm precisely what you want to accomplish. To make your goal achievable, make it specific and realistic. For example, if you're suffering from extreme back pain right now, you probably wouldn't set a goal to run a marathon next weekend. In that instance, a more realistic goal might be to walk for 15 minutes by next weekend.

Also, make sure you set a date to accomplish your goal. It's been said that a goal without a date is simply a wish. When you set a date, however, you will be more likely to work toward achieving your goal a step at a time. The progress you make will fuel you to continue each day, bringing you closer and closer to making your goal a reality.

Exercise

Exercise is as important when you're hurt or in pain as it is when you're healthy and pain free. Exercising can be as basic as walking, which will help get your blood flowing, keep your muscles flexible and strong, and get your heart circulating. Start small if you must, and make a goal to increase the length of your walk as you are able.

Water exercises are also excellent choices for those suffering back pain. Swimming, water aerobics, or water walking are all great because water decompresses the spine. When you're under water, gravity is eliminated, thus providing you with less resistance and relief.

While exercise is important to our overall health, as well as our healing process, it's important not to overdo it. Choose exercises that build the muscles that are weak, and be careful not to further stretch muscles that are already weak. Use Muscle Balance Therapy to identify the muscles that you want to focus on and select exercises which target those muscles.

CHAPTER 12

LIFESTYLE CHANGES THAT HELP BEAT PAIN

The more severe the pain or illness, the more severe will be the necessary changes. These may involve breaking bad habits, or acquiring some new and better ones.
Peter McWilliams

Since back pain is most commonly caused by imbalances in the body, several of the remaining chapters in this section will focus on body-based solutions. After that, we'll shift to solving mind- and diet-based problems. Your back pain is caused by a combination of factors, so I recommend you review each of these chapters to understand all the approaches that may be contributing to your suffering.

Finally, in the last section of the book, you'll find action plans for each type of back pain. These will tell you which treatment approaches to use in which order for each specific type of back pain and will refer to the treatments outlined in the next few chapters.

But first, we'll look at how simple lifestyle changes can be one of the easiest ways to alleviate back pain. Below are six key tips to get you started.

Tip #1:
Use Your Body Symmetrically

Because so many of us are either left- or right-handed, we tend to use one side of our bodies more than the other. This strengthens some muscles and leaves others underdeveloped and weak.

To create a better balance throughout the body—and better support for the spine and the back—start using both sides. If you normally lift your child with your right arm, for example, or balance her on your right hip, try lifting her with your left arm and balancing her on your left hip. Bend your knees when lifting her and never carry her for too long on just one side. Get used to shifting and using more of your muscles.

If you regularly carry a wallet or cell phone in your back pocket, remove it when you sit down. Even a slim model will tilt your hips to one side, which can lead to dysfunctional postures and muscle imbalances. You want to sit with a square, straight-on posture, so keep your back pockets empty.

Carrying a purse, diaper bag, or shoulder bag on one shoulder causes you to tilt and bend to compensate, straining your spine. It also forces the muscles on the carrying side to work harder than the ones on the other side. If you need to carry some sort of purse or bag on your shoulder, be sure to frequently switch, so both shoulders are worked equally. Or better yet, use a backpack that balances the load evenly.

If you're a regular traveler, you may want to invest in a wheeled laptop case, so you can keep the weight off your shoulders completely. Moms also can benefit from these types of wheeled suitcases, as they're a lot easier to carry around than a heavily loaded diaper bag.

Just as we tend to favor one side over the other, most of us lean forward more than we lean backward. Reading, driving, working at the computer, walking, running, cycling, writing, gardening... almost all activities require us to lean forward somewhat. Very few require that we lean backward. This weakens and stretches the muscles in our upper back, rounding the shoulders and tilting the neck forward and down.

This is such a chronic problem—probably the most common contributing factor to back pain—that I've devoted an entire later chapter to the topic, called Muscle Balance Therapy.

Tip #2:
Make Your Work Area
Posture Friendly

So many of us work at the computer these days. It's critical that we adjust the workspace so it encourages good posture. If your computer screen is positioned too low, you'll tend to look down at it, which fosters a forward neck and head posture. Bring it up to eye level.

What about your mouse? If it's too far forward and you have to reach to get it, again, you're pushing your body into a forward slump. Bring the mouse and keyboard back to where you can comfortably reach them or move your chair forward.

Make sure you have a good ergonomic chair, one that supports your back and fits your height and body structure, and preferably one with armrests. Wrist rests on your keyboard are also a good idea, as they help support the weight of your hands. Position the screen and the keyboard directly in front of you, so you don't have to rotate your neck or lower back. When typing, your fingers should rest easily on the keyboard with your elbows bent at 90-degree angles.

Don't forget to get up at least once an hour to walk around, stretch, and loosen up. Get a glass of water, take a walk outside, perform a handful of stretches, or visit with a colleague—anything to get your body moving.

Watch this free video to learn how to make
your work environment back friendly
www.losethebackpain.com/backpainnetwork

Tip #3:
Use a Telephone Headset

If you aren't doing so already, use an earpiece or a headset when talking on the phone. Avoid wedging the phone between your ear and your shoulder, as this puts extra strain on your back. Speakerphones are also good alternatives.

Tip #4:
Make Your Car Seat
Posture Friendly

Many of the same principles that apply to working at the computer also apply to driving. Make sure your lower back is well-supported. If your seat doesn't provide enough support, get a cushion or orthopedic-type support. The back of the seat should be slightly reclined, and the seat should be set at such a height that your hips are level with or slightly higher than your knees. Make sure you don't have to reach too far for the steering wheel or pedals. Your hands should rest comfortably on the wheel, without forcing your shoulders forward.

Above all, on long trips, stop, get out, walk, and stretch frequently.

Tip #5:
Use Posture Support Devices

While having good posture is essential to having less back pain, poor posture is usually a sign of two things. The first is imbalanced muscles, which we'll discuss in the chapter on Muscle Balance Therapy, and the second is using non-ergonomically designed devices—chairs, desks, keyboards, phones, etc.

It's important to realize that poor posture is not the problem—it's just the most visible sign of the problem. In almost all cases, poor posture is caused by muscle imbalances that make it nearly impossible to maintain and hold good posture.

Since you may not have the ability to easily modify the chair or car seat you use on a daily basis, using a posture support device can help improve your posture and relieve pressure points automatically—making a poor seat much better.

The most common posture support device to consider is a back support cushion. At a minimum, it should support your spine's natural "S" curve (as viewed from the side, not the back), particularly in the lumbar, or lower back area, of your spine.

Better back support cushions not only support good posture along your entire spine but include features such as anatomical contours to minimize direct pressure on the spine and even massage action to help relieve back muscle tension and improve circulation.

Another type of posture support device to consider is a back orthotic. Similar to how you walk on orthotics worn in shoes for foot support, you sit on a back orthotic placed on your seat which helps redistribute your weight in a manner that takes pressure off your spine, joints and ligaments while encouraging proper posture while sitting.

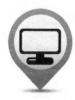

Learn more about the posture support
devices I recommend at:
www.losethebackpain.com/cushion

Tip #6:
For Women: Limit the Use and
Height of High Heels

High heels will make any back pain problem worse. They shorten the calf muscles, change your center of gravity, force you to overarch your back to keep from falling forward, pinch nerves, create trigger point stress areas, and more.

If you have to wear heels, try to stay with those that are two inches or less and limit the number of hours you wear them. As I've often said, pain is a message. If it hurts to wear heels, that's a message you may not want to ignore. And seriously, do you really "have to" wear them? It's your body and your choice.

These are all general recommendations for eliminating the most detrimental physical lifestyle habits that contribute to back pain and make existing back pain problems much worse.

In the next chapter, you'll learn what you can do to improve a common problem for back pain sufferers—get a good night's sleep.

CHAPTER 13

SLEEP WITHOUT PAIN

*A good laugh and a long sleep are the best
cures in the doctor's book.*
Irish Proverb

It's recommended that adults get seven to eight hours of sleep every night, but a third of all Americans are lucky if they catch six hours of sleep. For those who suffer from back pain, the percentage is even higher. Tossing and turning, they spend the entire night trying to get comfortable as they watch the precious minutes tick by.

Lack of sleep leaves us more than tired, irritable, and unable to function at our best—it actually can create health issues, including heart problems. It's also been suggested that sleep deprivation can cause inflammation. That's bad news for those with back pain, who might already be fighting inflammation associated with their back problem or injury.

Even if you can get to sleep, pain affects the quality of sleep you get. In order for the body to rejuvenate itself, which begins after you fall asleep, you need a period of deep sleep—a slumber that's difficult to achieve if you're tossing and turning all night. In this case, it's not how much sleep that you're getting that's the problem, but rather the inability to get the restful sleep that your body and mind need.

Why You Can't Sleep

Sleep—we need it and we love it. And when we don't get enough, it leaves us weary and energy deprived. The inability to get a good night of sleep is one of the biggest complaints among back pain sufferers. That's because there are many factors which are preventing them from enjoying some good shut eye, some of which actually contribute to their pain.

The bed or mattress. There are countless types of mattresses, from inflatable, adjustable ones, traditional mattresses built around a spring system, and even foam mattresses that mold to the body's contours. We've all seen the commercials for them, starring smiling men and women who wake up bright and shiny after a good night's sleep. Their hair isn't even out of place—your clue that they didn't toss and turn all night long.

Which one of these mattresses is right for you? Each person is different, and each person's pain is different. Therefore, the way any one person will respond to a particular mattress will be different than the next. In the past, it's been widely accepted that those with back pain should sleep on a firm mattress. However, a study of more than 300 adults who had chronic lower back pain found less pain and more improvement for those who slept on a medium-firm mattress. So, it appears comfort is a consideration in choosing your mattress. Firmer is not always better.

The type of mattress you choose can also depend on the cause of your back pain. People with sciatica require less flexion, so a firm mattress is often the best choice for them and their back pain. On the other hand, those with spinal stenosis do receive relief from mattresses that offer flexion. So a softer mattress would probably make them more comfortable. The large number of people who suffer from lower back pain are more likely to sleep better on a medium-firm mattress, although that's certainly not true in all cases.

Aging. The process of growing older does affect our sleep patterns. As we age, the body's production of some hormones decline, usually resulting in fewer hours of sleep.

Illness, Injury, or Pain. While pain can make us want to sleep, it doesn't help us sleep. Pain is a sleep blocker, which can keep us awake for long, tiring hours. This pain results in both lack of sleep and poor quality sleep, both of which leave us exhausted and less able to endure pain and restore our good health.

Stress. Minds that are riddled with worry and anxiety cannot rest. They don't shut off even when we're tired or asleep. Stress keeps our minds spinning and our eyes open, and when we finally do sleep, it's usually a bad night's sleep that serves to create more stress the next day.

Regardless of the reason, there are some things you can do to sleep better and longer, without the need to take prescription medication or sleep aids. Most of these are natural and are beneficial regardless of the cause of your pain or the reason why you can't sleep.

#1: Turn off the television

The TV is not a sleep aid. On the contrary, it's a cause of sleep disturbances. TV shows and commercials are meant to stimulate, which will work to counter sleepiness. That's why it's a good idea not to watch TV before you go to bed. And if you watch TV while you're in bed, turn it off! Reprogram your mind so it knows that the bed is for sleeping.

#2: Try a different pillow or mattress

If your mattress and pillows are old, it's time to go shopping. Mattresses and pillows age gradually, meaning we don't realize how much support they've lost over time. Find a good mattress that offers the support you need. Make sure you try it out—spend a few minutes lying on it at the store. Ask about the benefits of each one and get to know how they're constructed. If you can, opt for a mattress that has provided you with a good night's sleep when you were at a hotel or visiting friends or relatives. Above all, try to purchase from a store that offers a trial for a week or longer.

#3: Avoid caffeine

Coffee, tea, cola products, and even chocolate contain caffeine, which is a common culprit in sleep deprivation. If you can't avoid them altogether, limit their intake to mornings only and then in very small amounts.

#4: Listen to relaxing music

Instead of turning on the TV, try listening to relaxing music or a CD that feeds relaxing sounds, like ocean waves or babbling brooks, into your bedroom. The sound is soothing and peaceful, which just might be the ticket to lull you into a good night's sleep.

#5: Create a ritual that signals your mind that it's time to sleep

Starting tonight, create a ritual that is conducive to sleep. Help your body to unwind and prepare for sleep following this ritual every night at the same time and place. Your ritual might include soaking in a warm bath, meditation, yoga, or stretching exercises. Over time, your body will begin to recognize this time as preparation for sleep.

#6: Acupuncture

Some people have enjoyed good results at improving sleep from acupuncture. If the other methods listed here don't work for you, you might want to give it a try.

#7: Try a natural sleep aid

If you've exhausted the other methods and still can't sleep, a natural sleep aid might work. I don't recommend prescription or over-the-counter sleep aids, because many are addictive and have risky side effects, especially if taken for long periods of time. Instead, I suggest that you might want to try a safer alternative—a natural sleep aid.

While there are a number of natural sleep aids on the market, I've found they limit their formulas to one or a small handful of natural sleep aids. Worse, they often use unnatural fillers which can cause unintended side effects. I also found sleep aids with good ingredients often tended to work less effectively than they could due to low absorption.

That's why I partnered with a company to develop a natural sleep aid supplement combining 10 effective, natural sleep aids into a formula called Sleepzyme®. Not only does it eliminate fillers, it adds a digestive enzyme blend designed to boost absorption of the key ingredients so you can actually get to sleep.

If you're interested in trying an effective natural sleep aid supplement without unnatural fillers you can learn more about Sleepzyme® at **www.sleepzyme.com**.

CHAPTER 14

MAKE TRAVEL PAIN FREE

It is amazing how much crisper the general experience of life becomes when your body is given a chance to develop a little strength.
Frank Duff

Whether you're planning a yearly getaway to your favorite vacation spot or you're a daily commuter, traveling can place additional stressors on your back, legs, neck and shoulders. If you have back pain, travel can be difficult at best. Seats in buses, trains, cars, and planes aren't intended to provide the support needed for long hours of use. Often, they're too hard or simply not sized proportionately to your body frame. It doesn't take long in an uncomfortable seat before you begin to feel that familiar muscle strain or soreness.

The following simple tips can help you reduce or avoid back pain when traveling.

#1: Avoid stress by planning ahead

Stress contributes to and enhances pain. Reduce the amount of stress by making sure you plan ahead. Get permission and recommendations from your physician beforehand, if necessary, and make sure everything is organized and ready for your trip. Pack your bags a few days before the trip and load your suitcases into the car the night before. Shop for wardrobe items and needed supplies in advance, as well. This will reduce stress-related muscle cramps and back pain from exertion right before your trip.

If you can do anything online, do it—this includes shopping, reserving your airline ticket, and arranging for car rental or transportation when you arrive at your destination. Check your luggage at the curb so you don't have to carry it any more than necessary.

#2: Pack light

Heavy bags can aggravate back pain and strain your muscles and joints if you're not used to the physical exertion. Make things easier on yourself by using a suitcase with wheels and a handle for rolling it.

Use a few smaller bags instead of stuffing everything into one large suitcase which will be difficult for you to carry up stairs, lug around from place to place, and lift into and out of the car.

If heavy luggage is necessary, eliminate the opportunity for it to cause you back strain by taking advantage of the services of the airport baggage handler, taxi driver, and hotel bellhop.

#3: Use back and neck supports

Your lower back and neck can suffer if the seat doesn't provide enough support or if it doesn't support your body frame adequately. A good lumbar support pillow will make your seat more comfortable and add critical support for your lower back.

Avoid neck strain with a neck support pillow. Inflatable travel pillows for head support are inexpensive, lightweight, and are easy travel companions. Gone are the days where all airlines offered a pillow to every passenger, so it's always a good idea to bring one with you.

It may be more expensive, but the extra legroom found in business or first class may be worth it for your comfort. This is especially true if you have a long flight.

#4: Stretch

During long plane or train trips, be sure to get up and move around as frequently as possible, preferably every hour. Stand up, stretch, twist, and bend to ensure muscles throughout your body get refreshed.

Moving your muscles this way stimulates blood flow, bringing important nutrients and oxygen to tired muscles. Remember, simply holding the same position for extended periods is a major cause of muscle imbalances and lower back pain.

If you can manage just a few minutes of movement and stretching every hour, it will help prevent soft tissues in your lower back from stiffening and aching.

#5: Remain well hydrated

You can easily avoid dehydration, a common cause of back pain when traveling, if you remember to drink enough water during long trips.

Fluids are necessary to keep your body cool, your blood moving, your muscles supple and your tendons relaxed and pain free. Nothing replenishes the fluid in your body like good old water.

You can reduce your chance of back pain on long trips by avoiding tea, coffee, and alcohol, which can secretly leave you dehydrated.

Quick Remedies for Back Pain Relief While Traveling

If you experience back pain while traveling, fill a plastic bag with ice and apply it to the painful area. A cold pack is one of the fastest ways to get relief and reduce inflammation.

Hot packs and heat wraps can provide hours of comfort during lengthy trips, too. You might find it helpful to alternate heat and ice at 10 to 15 minute intervals, especially if you're experiencing muscle spasms.

Be sure to pack along a natural pain relief cream that can offer fast relief from unexpected pain.

Vacation Friendly Destinations
for Back Pain Sufferers

Lastly, when you're choosing a destination and making accommodations, choose one that's back pain friendly. Make note of the layout of the land, as well as the design of the hotel, house, or resort. Choose a vacation destination where it'll be easy for you to get around. Clearly you're likely to be more comfortable walking on flat ground rather than climbing hills; you're also likely to want your accommodations to have an elevator if you'll be staying on an upper level.

When you reach your destination, take a moment to relax in a bath or shower, letting water work its miracles on your tight muscles. Consider getting a massage from an on-site masseuse, but be sure to let him or her know of any specific medical issues in advance such as back surgeries you've had.

Schedule your vacation activities to allow plenty of time for rest and stretch breaks. Get in the pool while on vacation—water play is wonderful for an aching back.

Obviously, use common sense. Horseback riding and thrilling adventure rides might not be a preferred activity. Avoid activities that are likely to cause back pain or strain so you'll feel good enough to enjoy the rest of your vacation back pain free.

Now that we've reviewed some simple lifestyle changes to minimize back pain and its impact on your sleep and travel plans, we'll turn our attention to therapeutic solutions for your back pain. In the next few chapters, we'll talk about three different types of therapy that work for back pain caused by problems within the body. We'll discuss what each therapy does, when it's useful (and when it's not), for whom it's intended, and why it works.

CHAPTER 15

MUSCLE BALANCE THERAPY

*The breaking wave and the muscle as it contracts
obey the same law. A delicate line gathers the
body's total strength in a bold balance.*
Dag Hammarskjold

In this chapter, you'll learn how Muscle Balance Therapy works, when it works (and doesn't), and why it works. In the following chapters, I'll tell you about other proven treatment approaches, as well.

Later, in Part III, I'll provide action plans that address specific back pain conditions (sciatica, herniated disc, etc.). They'll tell you which therapies you should use and—if more than one therapy is needed—which combinations will be most effective for your particular condition.

What is Muscle Balance Therapy?

Muscle Balance Therapy is an innovative approach to eliminating back pain (and just about any other ailment) by addressing the imbalances in your muscles. In essence, it attempts to reverse the process that created the pain in the first place and bring your body back to a more neutral, properly aligned or "balanced" state.

The Muscle Balance Therapy approach begins by assessing the strength and flexibility of your muscle pairs—in your hips, pelvis, spine, and throughout the body. The idea is to find out which muscles are strong and which are weak, which are tight and which are more flexible, and which may be overworked or shortened.

Since these various imbalances stress joints, other muscles, and ligaments, the goal of the therapy is to rebalance the muscles— so that each muscle pair is as close to "normal" as possible. By evening out the muscle tension between the left and right sides of the body as well as between the front and back, the body supports the spine more evenly, automatically improving posture, allowing vertebrae to move back into position, and taking pressure off irritated nerves and muscles—thereby eliminating back pain.

Find out how Muscle Balance Therapy can
make you pain free in this free video!
www.losethebackpain.com/muscleimbalances

How Do I Determine If I Have Muscle Imbalances?

Well, the fact is that we all have muscle imbalances, but the key is to identify which ones you have. The good news is that this is something anyone can do, and it requires no special equipment or training. While there are experts, like me, who can perform very thorough evaluations, the fact is that you can identify the major imbalances on your own.

First, you perform several simple self-assessments, which help you to pinpoint the exact muscle imbalances you have. The assessments consist of stretches and exercises designed to test muscle strength and flexibility, visual evaluation of your posture using a mirror and photographs, and recording your results and findings.

Once you identify the physical dysfunctions you have and the muscle imbalances that are responsible, you then perform a very specific muscle rebalancing, stretching, and strengthening program. The idea is to strengthen those muscles that are overly weak, compared with the opposing muscles that form the muscle pair. Similarly, for those muscles that are tighter than their counterparts (i.e., shorter, with a smaller range of motion), you'd want to perform specific stretching exercises to correct the imbalance.

Determining muscle imbalances is such a visual exercise that a thorough assessment needs to include a series of photographs to evaluate your posture from the front, back, and both sides. If you were to look at pictures of how you normally stand, you'd be able to see many of the clues that I'll point out that serve as evidence of certain types of postural dysfunctions and muscle imbalances.

Finally, your assessment should include an evaluation of your history to determine any other areas of your life that might be contributing to your pain. All in all, the entire process will take approximately 30 minutes to an hour. Once you have completed the assessment, you'll feel confident that you have identified the imbalances and dysfunctions that you'll need to address.

In a moment, I'll share with you how you can assess yourself in the comfort of your own home.

Are These Muscle Imbalances Really That Important?

You want to pinpoint the muscles that are out of balance for two reasons: first, to determine which muscles are too weak, so you know how to strengthen and rebalance them; and second, to determine which muscles are overly strong (relative to the opposing muscles), so you can temporarily avoid strengthening them even more—which would make your back pain worse.

The problem of making strong muscles even stronger and tighter often occurs in people who have a single type of exercise they like to do over and over again. Someone who loves to do push-ups (making the chest muscles strong and tight), for example, but hates to do rows (which strengthen the opposing back muscles) would wind up with one type of muscle imbalance.

Another example is someone who rides a bicycle religiously but doesn't perform any opposing exercises. Cycling increases the strength of your quadriceps (the big upper leg muscles on the fronts of your thighs). But if you overdevelop these muscles without strengthening their opposing pairs—your hamstrings on the backs of your upper legs—this, too, will create or worsen muscle imbalances.

Incidentally, this is why general exercise and stretching has limited benefit when it comes to back pain. It's far more effective to exercise and stretch only the portions of the muscle pairs that need it.

How to Use Muscle Balance Therapy to Finally Get Lasting Relief

Properly diagnosing your muscle imbalances requires a step-by-step process that is known only to a small number of health care practitioners. Unfortunately, it's difficult to find out which practitioners understand the principles behind it.

To make life easier for back pain sufferers, I've created a Muscle Balance Therapy self-treatment kit.

This kit includes a video training program that shows you how your body should be moving when it's well-balanced. It includes reference photographs of how every major part of your body should look when sitting, standing, and walking. This allows you to compare your muscle-balance levels to those displayed on the videos and in the photographs—making it easy to isolate what's causing your back pain.

Several videos show you exactly what the different postural dysfunctions look like in action. Unfortunately, video material can't be conveyed very easily in the written format of a book. Once you see the various dysfunctions and compare them to how your body stands, sits, and walks, you'll be able to accurately assess your own condition.

The other critical thing that the videos show you is the proper way to implement the corrective stretches and exercises. This allows you to see what an imbalanced body looks like, how to fix it, and what your body should look like after you're done.

The Lose the Back Pain® System has been used by more than 70,000 people in more than 120 countries. You can learn more about this proven system by visiting my website at **www.losethebackpain.com/getstarted.**

Take Your Situation Seriously

Once you've determined your muscle imbalances and started the targeted exercises to address them (you'll find these in the videos included with the system), you'll start to feel better quickly. Within days you'll probably notice some relief, and if you continue the corrective exercises, you'll find your body making steady progress and your back pain fading.

This program has been successful at helping so many with back pain that I urge you to give it a try for lasting back pain relief. You can even download the digital version from the URL above if you want to get started immediately.

Muscle imbalances are one of the biggest factors in creating back pain—especially nerve-based back pain. However, there's another little known cause of pain called trigger points. In the next chapter, you'll learn more about trigger points, how they develop and cause pain, and most important, how to effectively treat them.

CHAPTER 16

TRIGGER POINT THERAPY

*Our real problem, then, is not our strength today;
it is rather the vital necessity of action today to
ensure our strength tomorrow.*
Dwight D. Eisenhower

As I've mentioned, there are two types of back pain: pain caused by an irritated nerve, known as nerve-based back pain, and tissue pain, which can be caused by muscle imbalances, as well as dietary and emotional imbalances.

But another little-known cause exists—trigger points, or knots, within a muscle.

In this chapter, I'll discuss trigger point therapy, the most effective treatment approach for most cases of knotted-muscle pain.

Keep in mind that if you suffer from both nerve- and tissue-based back pain, trigger point therapy will solve only part of your problem.

In addition, while trigger point therapy is great at getting rid of the knots that cause back pain, it doesn't prevent those knots from forming in the first place.

In severe cases of tissue-based pain, you'll also want to prevent the creation of knots—or more typically, prevent preexisting trigger point areas from flaring up. To do this, you'll need to focus on changes in lifestyle, particularly dealing with problems in the mind (e.g., stress) and diet, which we will cover later in this section.

What is a Trigger Point?

A trigger point is essentially a small, hard, painful knot within a muscle. Imagine a muscle as a handful of spaghetti, with each straight, hanging noodle representing a muscle fiber.

In a healthy muscle, all the fibers are long and even, like spaghetti, or like the hairs on the bow of a violin. A trigger point causes an unhealthy contraction, so that some of those fibers twist, or seize up, into a knot.

When a knot appears in a muscle, it causes pain for two reasons. First, the muscle loses access to the nutrients in the blood, and second, without healthy circulation passing through, toxins tend to build up in the contracted area.

The muscle typically shortens as well, just like a strand of rope shortens when you tie a few knots in the middle of it. (This often restricts the range of motion and flexibility in the affected area.)

You can feel a trigger point. If you massage another person, when your fingers run over hard knots under the skin, they are usually trigger points.

To be certain, check for the same hard point on the opposite side of the body. If you find one near the right shoulder blade, for instance, check near the left shoulder blade. If you find a similar hard spot, it's probably a bone, but if you don't, that first one was probably a trigger point.

These little knots are also typically sensitive to touch. So if you press on it and the person yelps, you can bet you've hit a trigger point.

Trigger points also can cause general pain, tightness or restriction of movement, false heart pain, headaches, neck and jaw pain, tennis elbow, joint pain, restless legs, and numbness in the hands and feet.

Do trigger points have you knotted up?
If so, watch this free video demonstrating
how to self-treat trigger points at
www.losethebackpain.com/triggerpoints

Trigger Points Can Cause Many Other Problems

Once you have a trigger point, or several of them, you will likely alter the way you move, sit, or stand to instinctively protect yourself. Moving a certain way causes you pain, so you try to avoid it.

At the same time, the muscle is contracting to protect itself. Unfortunately, all this makes the problem worse, as then your body begins to adopt crooked postures that tighten other muscles, leading to additional or worsening existing muscle imbalances.

This is one reason some people have both nerve-based back pain caused by muscle imbalances and tissue-based back pain caused by a knot or trigger point within a single muscle.

Such postures then put pressure on joints and ligaments, further restricting your activities. This vicious cycle can come full circle, creating more trigger points and starting the process all over again.

You can see how this quickly leads to lower back pain if you have trigger points anywhere around the lower body.

They also can cause upper back pain, typically between the shoulder blades or at the base of the neck, as these muscles often are overworked, tense, or used in a dysfunctional way due to the muscle imbalances.

Of course, pain in the upper back, shoulders, and neck often lead to headaches, as well.

To live a pain free life, it's critical to treat and relieve trigger points as quickly and thoroughly as possible.

What Causes Trigger Points?

While there are many factors that contribute to the development of trigger points, one of the most common is blood circulation that's too slow or restricted.

One major cause is stress. When you're experiencing too much stress, you tend to tense your muscles (reducing blood circulation in those muscles), drink too little water (reducing the blood volume available to clear out toxins in the muscles), eat too much unhealthy food (causing inflammation that makes trigger points swell), and forget to move around and stretch (reducing blood circulation in your muscles).

These behaviors lead to shallow breathing, which delivers too little oxygen to your muscles. Your tenseness and anxiety lead to decreased blood flow—that stagnation or "too slow" we mentioned in earlier chapters.

Without adequate blood flow, the muscle cells in the trigger point areas of your body are unable to activate the relaxation response that makes the trigger point disappear or at least go dormant. The mechanism that allows muscle cells to "let go" requires the oxygen and energy provided by good blood circulation.

Trigger points also can occur as a result of muscle trauma (from car accidents, falls, sports- and work-related injuries, etc.), muscle strain from repetitive movements or strenuous exercise, muscle imbalances, sitting for long periods, nutritional deficiencies, and more. Unfortunately, once you have a trigger point, it tends to undergo a self-reinforcing cycle—which means it sticks around for a while.

Active and Inactive Trigger Points

Most of us are walking around with trigger points. Just the stresses of living can create them in our bodies over time.

Whether or not they cause us pain hinges on whether or not they are "active" at any particular time.

Active trigger points are the ones that feel painful. Inactive ones don't radiate pain but may still exist as knots and feel painful if you apply pressure to them.

After a trigger point has healed, that area of the muscle tends to have a good memory. The trigger point has "branded" it, so to speak, so the next time you experience stress, overwork certain muscles, or fail to drink enough water, that muscle can contract again in the same place, activating the same trigger point as before.

Imagine a ceramic coffee cup. Let's say that one day you accidentally drop it and break the handle. No worries; you use some superglue and seal the handle back on. But that handle now has an old injury. You can bet that if you were to drop the cup again, the handle would break in the very same place.

Trigger points act the same way, particularly if they aren't healed completely. They tend to return again and again, whenever the body is under stress. The best approach is to adopt healing solutions and lifestyle habits that keep trigger points relaxed and dormant—and keep new ones from developing.

Trigger Points and "Referred" Pain

I've been emphasizing all along how important it is to look beyond the pain you're experiencing so you can address the cause of that pain. Here's another reason why: Trigger points can cause pain in other parts of the body.

We call this "referred" pain. It's as if the trigger point "refers" its pain to some other muscle or area of the body, saying, "Here, you take this message to the brain."

For example, you could be feeling pain in your hips, buttocks, or down your legs, when the actual trigger point is located in your lower back. Trigger points also can refer pain to other trigger points along the same nerve pathways.

So, if your health practitioner is not educated in seeking out the cause of the pain, she may simply focus on the location of that pain—your legs, for example—while ignoring the fact that the trigger point in your lower back is causing it. That's unfortunate, because then any treatments she implements will only partially (if at all) help the condition.

Another example is pain in your arm, mid-back, or neck. These all could be caused by a trigger point in your shoulder. Any treatment that fails to address your shoulder problem is going to be unsuccessful. Therefore, it's important to find the trigger points, wherever they are, and heal them, one by one.

So What is Trigger Point Therapy?

Trigger point therapy is a method by which steady, sustained pressure is applied to the "knotted" area. Such pressure gradually encourages the muscle fibers to relax and release, loosening the twisted places. Since muscles that have trigger points are typically too tight and too short, trigger point therapy encourages elongation and relaxation.

As the fibers return to a more healthy shape, they let loose all the pent-up toxins that had been trapped there, returning them to the bloodstream where they can be washed away. Blood flow increases through the area, encouraging waste removal and healing. Eventually, muscle spasms disappear, tenseness goes away, and the muscle returns to more normal function.

This process also creates an overall body release, or "sigh of relief," reducing the pain signals to the brain and alerting your system to restore itself.

This kind of therapy is helpful for any type of back pain that originates in trigger points, which could include lower back pain, upper back pain, neck pain, any muscle-based pain, and fibromyalgia—

even some nerve-based pain like sciatica and herniated discs, if the muscles around the nerves are knotted up in trigger points.

Water is Essential to Healing

When you're undergoing treatment for trigger points, it's essential to drink a lot of water. Pressure on the knots in your muscles releases toxin buildup, which means those toxins then become more plentiful in your bloodstream. You need water to flush them out of the body.

Imagine hard water buildup in a humidifier or copper pipe. Once that buildup is broken down into smaller pieces, you need extra water to wash it away. Otherwise, it will continue to linger, perhaps even build up in other locations.

If you have a very severe case of trigger point-caused back pain, don't be surprised if, after your first one or two treatments, you feel a little ill. If you had a lot of toxin buildup in your muscles, those toxins will flood your body once released, which can have a physical effect on you. You're essentially releasing months' worth of garbage from your muscles into your bloodstream—ultimately allowing your kidneys to convert the waste into urine. Drink plenty of water to ensure that the toxin levels don't get so high they make you feel sick.

Three Trigger Point Solutions

I'm now going to talk about three solutions to trigger points and the pros and cons of each: 1) the handheld pressuring device, 2) trigger point massage therapy, and 3) the self-treatment platform.

1. The Handheld Pressuring Device

A popular item on the market is the handheld self-massager, usually a plastic device shaped like a hook or cane, with rounded "balls" on either end and on additional "steps" along the straight edge. These rounded sections are meant to be used to apply pressure to your trigger points. Two examples of this type of device are the "Theracane" and the "Backnobber."

Similar to a back scratcher, this device requires you to do your own work on the areas that are causing you pain. Essentially, you hold the device in your hand, maneuver it to reach the trigger point (usually in your back), and apply pressure, typically in an area no larger than a quarter. The shape of the device gives you some leverage, but you're using your muscles to do the work. You move the ball back and forth across the trigger point, wiggling it a bit to get deeper into the muscle.

The idea is that, after several repeated applications of pressure with the device, your trigger points will loosen up, release toxins, and gradually relieve you of pain.

The good thing about this solution is that it puts you in charge of your own relief. You have the device in your home, where you can use it at your convenience. It's fairly economical—a one-time purchase—and can be used as often as you need without additional cost.

What concerns me with devices like these is that one, they can be awkward to use, and two, they have the potential to make your situation worse. Basically, unless you're using the device on your legs, you're asking the same muscles that may be experiencing pain to fix the problem.

For example, if you have a trigger point in the muscle behind your shoulder blade, you have to use that same muscle to maneuver the device and apply pressure to the trigger point. First of all, it can be a little difficult to get the device where you want it. Second, you're contracting the injured muscle, and a muscle suffering from trigger points certainly doesn't need more contraction. It's like asking a person with a sprained ankle to walk himself to the hospital.

Using this device on any trigger point in any area of your back is going to require the same (or nearby) back muscles to work. If you're not careful, you could be creating more trigger points in muscles that are already overworked, shortened, and inflamed.

I recommend you try using a device like this and see how it works for you.

2. Trigger Point Massage Therapy

Trigger point massage can be a very effective therapy. It's a form of massage in which the practitioner applies deep pressure to isolated areas of your body—your trigger points.

First, you're lying down, resting, while the therapist works on your trigger points, so you don't have the problems that exist with the handheld pressuring device. Your back muscles are as relaxed as they can be, and the massage therapist commonly uses his elbow to apply vertical pressure on each trigger point.

Trigger point massage is different than regular massage. Instead of implementing longer, sloping movements that lightly pressure the length of your muscles, the therapist will apply targeted, firm, and sustained pressure (about 7 to 10 seconds) directly on the trigger point. At first, this probably won't feel very good. The trigger point is painful, and pressure will activate that pain—as well as release toxins—both of which can be uncomfortable.

However, if proper pressure is applied on a regular basis, eventually the trigger points will relax and release, and your pain will go away. The pressure physically forces blood circulation into the trigger point area, giving the muscle cells in the trigger point the oxygen and fuel needed to activate the relaxation mechanism.

Trigger point massage is a great solution. The only drawbacks are that it can get very expensive and can take up a considerable amount of your time. One treatment isn't going to do the trick. You need to go back several times to completely heal the trigger points—often at least weekly—and since this type of specialty massage typically costs

$60 to $100 per hour, it can add up in a hurry.

The number of visits it takes can depend on many things, including how long you've had the trigger point, how many you have, how effective the treatment is, and how consistently you receive the treatment. However, there are other solutions that work well, are actually more convenient, and cost much less.

3. Trigger Point Self-Treatment Platform

The most economical and effective method I've found for treating trigger points is to use a self-treatment platform. You use this treatment approach by lying down on a platform that has a number of soft, rubber-tipped pressure bumps on it. You configure this platform to match the trigger points on your back. For example, if you have a trigger point just under your right shoulder blade, you place a pressure bump on the platform in the position where your right shoulder will be when you lie down.

The idea is not to apply pressure to every part of your back, but only to the parts that have trigger points. You position the rubber-tipped pressure bumps where you need them and then lie down on top of them. Gravity takes over. Because the platform comes with pressure providers of different heights, you can choose the intensity of the pressure. Shorter providers give lighter pressure; longer ones, more intense pressure. This allows you to configure the platform to mirror the location and severity of the trigger points in your back.

There are several advantages to this sort of device. First, you're not requiring sore, irritated muscles to work harder in an effort to gain relief. Second, you're investing once in a device you can use for the rest of your life, so you're saving a significant amount of money. Third, you're putting yourself in charge of your relief, which means you can use the device when it's most convenient for you, and as often as you need, without a bunch of hassles.

Finally, it's the sort of solution that gives you immediate feedback.

When you lie on a trigger point, you'll know it, because of the sore, numb, or slightly painful reaction in the muscle. If you don't feel that reaction, you can adjust your position on the platform or adjust the pressure providers to a location that will be more effective. It's a very intuitive process that's easy to perform.

Conclusion

You can find more information on how to identify and treat trigger points, including a video demonstration of how to release trigger points on your own, on my website at **www.losethebackpain. com/triggerpoints.**

At this point, we've covered two types of body-based solutions: Muscle Balance Therapy and trigger point therapy. If you're suffering from nerve- or muscle-based pain because of tight, inflamed, over-worked, and knotted muscles, these two solutions may provide you with complete relief.

However, you also will likely benefit greatly from an additional treatment approach that I'll cover next—spinal decompression therapy.

CHAPTER 17

SPINAL DECOMPRESSION THERAPY

There are two ways of exerting one's strength:
one is pushing down, the other is pulling up.
Booker T. Washington

Two thousand years ago, Hippocrates, the "Father of Medicine," used the first form of spinal decompression therapy to help patients with back pain. Since that time, literally millions have used this simple technique to reduce or eliminate their pain. Yet, it's unlikely that your doctor has ever recommended it.

As I explained earlier, the fact is that most doctors just don't know about many of these natural or "alternative" treatments. And then there are some who will instantly dismiss them, either because of their simplicity or because of misinformation. Either way, millions of people suffer with back pain and never learn of these proven treatments.

Inversion therapy, the oldest, most well-known, and commonly used form of spinal decompression therapy, can be very effective for those who suffer from nerve-based back pain or sciatica—particularly, those with a herniated or bulging disc. It offers quick, reliable pain relief, as well as some long-term positive effects. Nearly everyone can benefit from inversion therapy, because even if a person doesn't have pain, the additional benefits are well worth the 3 to 5 minutes.

We'll discuss later under which circumstances and for how long you should use inversion therapy, as well as some alternative forms of spinal decompression therapy, but for now, let's review how and why inversion therapy works.

What is Inversion Therapy?

As the name states, inversion therapy actually "inverts" the body to an upside-down position. There are several ways this can be performed, but the most common is by using what's called an inversion table.

An inversion table sits on a swivel and is made for you to lie on. Think of a seesaw with a bed on it—only the midpoint of the seesaw is much higher, so if you lean all the way forward you're fully upright, and if you lean all the way back, you're upside down.

The idea behind inversion therapy is to reverse the effects of gravity. Since we live on Earth, we're all subjected to the force of gravity on a day-to-day basis. Our muscles and bones help us stand up against it, but over the years, it tends to wear us down a bit— particularly the spine, which is the center of our upright posture.

Spinal Compression

The spine is made up of a series of bones called vertebrae that are stacked one on top of the other. Between these bones are doughnut-shaped discs—gel-like structures that are filled mostly with water and serve as the body's shock absorbers.

We've talked about how muscle imbalances can create postural dysfunctions that pressure the spine, in essence "squishing" the discs in uneven ways. A combination of tight and weak muscles can literally tilt the stack of vertebrae too far in any direction, greatly increasing the stress on one side of any particular disc.

Imagine a balloon, for instance, one of those long ones that can be twisted into different shapes to make balloon animals. If you were to squish one side with your fist, all the air in the balloon would form a bulge at the other side. Keep pressing, and eventually you could force the other end of the balloon to burst.

Discs operate much the same way. As muscle imbalances—and gravity—apply uneven pressure on a disc, the disc bulges to one side. This is what happens in the case of a herniated disc. The disc has actually developed a hernia, or bulge, at one end. This bulge then often comes into contact with a nerve, which is what many doctors believe causes the sharp, radiating pain of this condition. Eventually, if the problem is not corrected, the disc can burst, losing its water content and its ability to absorb any shock at all.

Even if we don't have muscle imbalances adding to the issue, which we all do, gravity by itself creates a daily compression on our spines. You may not realize this, but as you go about your day, gravity presses down on your discs, causing the water inside them to slowly squeeze out. Measurements taken have shown that most people are slightly shorter at the end of the day than they were at the beginning— by as much as three-quarters of an inch!

Fortunately, the spinal discs reabsorb water while we sleep (as long as we're not dehydrated), so we start the day again at close to our regular height. However, over the years, our discs lose their ability to "re-inflate," so we grow a little shorter by the time we become seniors. (I imagine that's why we have the terms "little old lady" and "little old man.")

How Does Inversion Therapy Help?

Inversion therapy literally reverses the compression caused by gravity—and in part, muscle imbalances. In essence, it reverses the pressure on the spine that is a result of gravity and muscle imbalances. Instead of compressing your discs and making you shorter, inversion therapy—by allowing you to hang upside down—actually stretches the spine out, as well as the muscles supporting the spine and torso, giving the discs room to reabsorb fluids and move back into their proper positions—eliminating pressure on nearby nerves.

Download my comprehensive report,
Heal Your Body with Spinal Decompression,
on this back pain therapy free from:
www.losethebackpain.com/decompressionheals

Space Gives Injured Discs Room to Heal

With the increased spaces between the vertebrae that inversion therapy creates, discs are suddenly relieved of pressure and have room to breathe, so to speak. Even the slightest increase in spacing can create a mild suction, which can encourage a bulging disc to return to its normal position. In essence, space gives the disc the room it needs to heal.

If you picture again that balloon, it's like taking your fist off one end and allowing the air inside to fill up the entire area once again.

What does this mean to you? Pain relief. If a disc is pressing on a nerve, inversion therapy often will relieve that pressure, easing pain almost immediately.

According to many clinical studies, inversion therapy is one of the most effective and fastest ways to increase space between your vertebrae. I've actually had clients tell me that their back pain, pain that had plagued them for decades, totally disappeared with just a few minutes of inversion therapy.

Other cases completely reversed themselves with just a week of inversion therapy—10 minutes a day of hanging upside down. If you need to get back to work and you suspect a herniated disc could be the source of your pain, inversion therapy may be the best way to recover. (Just remember to address any other causes of your pain, as well!)

And in case you doubt the effectiveness of inversion therapy, a study conducted by Newcastle University found that back pain sufferers who underwent inversion therapy were 75 percent less likely to require back surgery!

Back Ease - An Alternative to Inversion Tables

Although specialized machines found in the offices of some doctors, chiropractors and physical therapists can provide spinal decompression without inversion, regular use can be costly. However, a new device called the Back Ease allows people to get many of the benefits of inversion therapy at home without inverting.

Those who are frail or weak often find the Back Ease a better option than inversion. This particular device is slightly better than traditional inversion tables at decompressing the lower spine. People who have herniated discs in that area may benefit from it because the device allows them to apply and increase the amount of traction targeted on the lower back, where it will provide them with the most relief.

You can learn more about the Back Ease online by going to: **www.losethebackpain.com/backease**.

The Many Other Benefits of Inversion Therapy

Though increasing space between the vertebrae through spinal decompression is one of the biggest benefits of inversion therapy, it's definitely not the only one. Let's take a look at several other benefits.

Improves circulation. Turning the body upside down, for your blood, is like taking a road that normally climbs uphill and making it go downhill. In other words, where the blood usually had to travel up, it now heads down, and vice versa. Suddenly it's easier for the blood to get to certain areas that are usually a challenge to reach— particularly the upper back, neck, and head. This makes it easier for some of the muscles and joints to get access to the nutrients and oxygen they need.

Lengthens muscles and ligaments. Inverting the body has a natural stretching effect on many of your muscles and ligaments. You can feel it while it's happening. Pitch yourself upside down for even a moment and you'll feel some of the muscles in your back, legs, and hips pulling toward the ground, which has a stretching effect. Since these muscles are usually pulled in the opposite direction by gravity, inversion therapy helps counteract that effect, pulling them in the other direction and increasing flexibility.

Relieves joints. Point the head toward the ground and, instantly, knee, hip, ankle, and other joints experience a gentle "opening." Similar to the way inversion therapy eases pressure on the spine, it does the same to weight-bearing joints that are typically loaded all the time, every day. With the absence of pressure, the joints get momentary relief, during which they, like the discs in the spine, gradually open up and "breathe." This effect can be felt for hours after the therapy, in joints that feel more springy and supple.

Improves posture. Though inversion therapy will not correct muscle imbalances, it may help a crooked spine to realign itself. By using the power of gravity to pull in the opposite direction, inversion therapy encourages the spine to resume its normal posture.

It's like pulling on the bottom of a wrinkled shirt to straighten it out. Gravity pulls the spine toward your head. Given enough time (through repeated treatments), the vertebrae can line back up. When you stand upright again, you'll feel the effects and enjoy better posture. If you combine this therapy with Muscle Balance Therapy, you'll be more likely to maintain that improved body position.

Maintains your height. We would all like to maintain our stature as we get older. Inversion therapy helps counteract the typical wearing down of the spine over the years, helping us avoid the shrinkage associated with old age. Discs that have been ground down over time get a "breather" and a chance to reabsorb fluid so they can regain their shock-absorbing capacity. It's these same discs that, when worn down, contribute to that hunched-back posture that plagues many older people.

Increases mental alertness. Some authorities believe that increasing oxygen and blood flow to the brain can help maintain mental sharpness. Since this is such an important goal for seniors—as evidenced by all the sales of mental-support supplements—such a benefit could be very welcome.

Helps in workout recovery. Running, cycling, and other aerobic activities can actively compress the spine, oftentimes in uneven ways. One-sided sports like tennis, racquetball, and golf can pull the spine out of alignment because of the repeated twisting motions. With regular inversion therapy, any misalignments between the vertebrae often are self-corrected.

Is It Safe?

Some people may have heard that inversion therapy can increase the chance of having a stroke. I think this is an unfortunate result of misinformation. Yes, there was a study published in 1983 by Dr. Steven A. Goldman in which he observed that inverted patients experienced an increase in blood pressure. The media jumped on the story, warning people that inversion therapy could lead to stroke.

What they didn't report as widely was that two years later Dr. Goldman recanted his position, stating, "New research shows that you are at no more of a stroke risk hanging upside down than if you are exercising right-side up." He said that the media's warnings about inversion therapy were "grossly inflated." Further research actually discovered that the body has built-in ways to prevent any damage from hanging upside down. Unfortunately, this news wasn't as exciting, so few people ever heard it, and many remained concerned about using this very beneficial treatment.

Of course, I recommend that you should be in basic good health if you're going to try inversion therapy. If you have high blood pressure, heart disease, an eye condition, are pregnant, or have had fusion surgery or a knee or hip replacement, you should check with your doctor before trying inversion therapy. However, research shows that this therapy is as safe as most daily activities. According to Roger Teeter, one of the pioneers in the field of inversion therapy, "In 25 years, I have never seen a case—published or unpublished—where inversion [therapy] caused a stroke." Plus, high blood pressure does not cause a stroke. High blood pressure is simply an indicator of a possible health problem that could lead to a stroke, much like a fever alerts you to sickness.

What's the Best Way to Do It?

Though "gravity boots" were popular in the 1980s, the most common way to invert today is by using an inversion table. There is a wide variety of them on the market. So what do you need to look for?

First, I recommend investing in a quality inversion table—one that's going to last and that has the proper safety features. There are a lot of companies making these, and many of them skimp on quality to bring their prices down. If you're hanging upside down, you want something that's going to support you, time after time. You don't want to save a few bucks just to land on your head! In fact, one manufacturer recently had to recall one of its models due to safety malfunctions.

Look for a table that's adjustable, safe, durable, and convenient for using in your home.

Adjustable. Your table should adjust to a variety of angles, from a slight downward tilt to full inversion, which puts you completely upside down. Adjusting ability is important because you want to give your body time to gradually adapt to being inverted. You may not want to hang completely upside down for a full 10 minutes the first time. Your body won't be used to it.

Instead, I typically recommend clients start at a gentle angle for a few minutes, then gradually increase it as they grow more comfortable. Adjustment ability also is helpful if you want to ease the blood flow to your head for a moment, then return to full inversion. So make sure you can control the angle of your equipment. You never have to fully invert unless you want to. As little as a 25° angle can give you near instant pain relief while only a 60° angle is needed to completely remove the load of gravity from your spine.

In addition, it's nice to have a table that can be used by people of varying heights. Once you have an inversion table in your home, don't be surprised if others in the family want to try it out.

Safe. I can't stress enough the importance of this quality. Make sure that whatever table you are investing in has been proven safe— preferably by an independent testing facility. Check to be sure that it can properly support your weight and that the footrests are adequately padded to avoid any injury to your ankles and feet.

Durable. I don't think I have to tell you that you don't want a plastic inversion table. Get one made of durable materials, preferably steel, that carries a long warranty. You'll be making an investment in a piece of equipment that you'll probably use the rest of your life, so do your research.

Convenient. Since you'll be using this in your home, you want it to be convenient. First, make sure that you can assemble it easily. It's very frustrating to get something into your home that you can't even put together. Second, if you have limited space, consider looking for a folding model so you can store it in a closet or under a bed if you want to.

In addition to these four things, I also recommend that you look for a table that comes with some customer support. A user's guide, a video guide, and telephone support all can come in really handy if you have questions. Without these things, you could end up frustrated if you're missing a part, for instance, or if you have questions about how long or how often to hang upside down.

A process that includes a gradual increase of the angle of inversion, as well as a gradual increase of time spent upside down, is best for relieving back pain. A good user's manual or video guide can help you set up such a process for yourself, increasing your odds of success.

Get more information about the inversion
table I use and recommend to all of my clients
at **www.losethebackpain.com/inversion**

Conclusion

We've now covered the main solutions to body-based back pain. In the next two chapters, we'll be discussing solutions to address the mind and diet.

CHAPTER 18

BALANCE YOUR EMOTIONAL STATE OF MIND

Just as your car runs more smoothly and requires less energy to go faster and farther when the wheels are in perfect alignment, you perform better when your thoughts, feelings, emotions, goals, and values are in balance.
Brian Tracy

In Chapter 7, I talked about how emotions and stress can contribute to back pain, as well as nearly every health ailment known to man. They can make muscles tight (contributing to muscle imbalances), decrease our oxygen supply, release hormones that trigger inflammation, and create trigger points in areas where we "hold" our stress—such as the shoulders and lower back—all leading to real physical pain.

Here are four tips to help ease stress and balance your emotional state of mind.

Tip #1:
Be Aware of the Emotional Component of Pain

Sometimes, just becoming aware of the cause of a problem can help you alleviate it. If stress and emotional upset are causing your back pain—and if you've been told there's nothing physically wrong with you—hearing that emotional imbalances can be real, concrete causes of physical pain can be a big relief. The pain isn't just "in your head." It's real pain that just happens (in some cases) to start from mental stress, strain, or trauma.

Not knowing why you have back pain is, well, stressful. It leaves you imagining some mysterious cause. This uncertainty creates more stress, which creates even more back pain, and the cycle repeats.

The good thing is that once you know that stress—and in some extreme cases, emotional trauma—also is causing or contributing to your back pain (in addition to the many other ways it may be impacting your life), you may take it seriously enough to address it.

Tip #2:
Reduce or Eliminate the
Negative Stress in Your Life

Most of us know this one. If we could just eliminate all the things causing us stress, we'd feel great! But who can do that, right?

I think we tend to dismiss this a little too quickly, though. Sometimes all it takes is a healthy dose of self-care. Give yourself permission to do what's best for you. For example, how many times do you say "yes" to someone you don't even like? How often do you take on extra tasks that do nothing to help you or the ones you love? Start there. Give yourself permission to say "no."

Next, look at the people around you. How much time do you spend around negative people? You know the ones. They're always complaining about something. Everything is bad; nothing is ever good. These people tend to rob us of our energy and well-being. Make it a point to stay away from them. If that's not possible (which is really just an excuse), keep your interactions short. You've got somewhere to go, a phone call to make, whatever.

If you can't get away from the person—a family member, for instance—try redirecting the conversation in a more positive direction.

If that doesn't work, erect an imaginary bubble around you to help avoid the negative energy. You may even want to confront the person. Explain your attempts to reduce your stress, and gently tell them that the negative conversation contributes to the problem. Suggest a more positive approach to life and maybe they'll respond. If not, and you feel that this person is really placing a heavy negative drain on you, you may want to consider separating this person from your life. Far too many people spend most of their lives in pain and being unhappy; don't be one of them.

Of course, our jobs can create a lot of stress in our lives. If you think yours is contributing to your back pain, consider a change. Changing careers solely to reduce back pain may not be practical for many people, but back pain combined with other factors (such as career unhappiness) might be enough to warrant an exploration of other occupations.

If a job change is just impossible at this point in time, explore ways to reduce your stress levels. Can you delegate more tasks to others? Can you take real lunch breaks, where you get away from the environment to somewhere that nourishes your spirit? How about talking to your supervisor to implement some changes? Hiring an assistant or an intern, perhaps?

Another thing that many people forget to think about is their living environment. Is yours comfortable and peaceful, allowing you to relax and refuel at the end of the day? Or do you find yourself more stressed at home than you are at work? Getting rid of clutter can do a lot to reduce stress. Have a "giveaway" day where you donate all the material things you don't need to charity. Creating some space in your home gives you room to breathe easier.

What about finances? In a tough economy, concern over finances can cause a lot of physical pain. Sometimes downsizing your lifestyle, and the bills that go with it, can provide instant stress relief. Again, back pain alone probably isn't enough of a reason to make major financial changes in your life, but it may tip the scales toward making changes.

In general, take a good look at your life—your job, your surroundings, your schedule, your friends and family—and find out what's nourishing and what's draining. Whenever possible, eliminate the draining factors.

Tip #3:
Get It Out

In Chapter 7, I also talked about how destructive repressed emotions are. For back pain, they're the most destructive. So no matter what kind of emotional stress you're under, it's important to get it out—in a healthy way. Stress, anxiety, and emotional trauma held within the body damage the body. Get the stress out of your system and the pain follows, too.

For the more severe cases of emotional trauma, such as death, divorce, abandonment, and abuse, the techniques for managing everyday stress may not be enough. One advanced technique is to write down the pent-up emotions you're feeling (the most common one is anger).

Use a pen and notepad, your computer, or even a voice recorder to get your emotions out. Start with feeling words like, "I'm angry about...," "I wish...," "I'm sorry for..." "I feel..." and other similar expressions to encourage emotional responses. Typically, these kinds of exercises help clear your head and release the pressure that emotions can create in the body.

For serious traumas that may have occurred in the past but that were never resolved, it's best to seek the assistance of a licensed therapist. Even if you're not sure such a trauma could be causing your back pain, if you've experienced something very difficult—a crime, childhood abandonment or abuse, rape, or other type of violence—it's paramount that you properly process the experience.

These deeply disturbing episodes can lodge themselves in your body and continue to cause pain for years. If you've suppressed the emotions surrounding these events, you may not be aware of the damage they're causing. Try a few visits with a reputable therapist and see if you notice an improvement in your back pain.

Some types of therapy you may want to consider are gestalt therapy, family constellation therapy, and hypnosis.

Tip #4:
Manage the Stress
You Do Have

Stress is not all bad. We need some stress in our lives to feel alive and excited about the future. If everything was calm and routine all the time, we'd get bored pretty quickly.

So, after you've eliminated all the stress you can, you must decide how to manage what remains.

One of the best ways I know to cope with stress is to exercise. It releases your body's natural feel-good endorphins, gives you energy, relieves pain, burns calories (potentially helping you to lose weight), and helps you live longer. There's really no end to the benefits of this powerful coping technique.

So make time in your daily schedule to move—first thing in the morning, as a break at midday (a lunchtime walk can do wonders), as a bridge between work and home life—however it works best for you. Get into the habit, and don't give that time away to anyone.

Resist the impulse to say, "Well, I can exercise tomorrow." If you were to meet a friend for a walk, you wouldn't easily cancel that, would you? Take the appointments you make with yourself just as seriously.

Another great way to reduce stress is through meditation. Taking 10 to 20 minutes a day to be still, breathe deep, and center your thoughts quiets both the mind and the body, reducing all the stress-induced changes that are so bad for your health. Many meditation techniques really emphasize slow, deep breathing— which is great for getting more oxygen into your muscle cells, reducing the likelihood of trigger points. It's also the exact opposite of the fast and shallow breathing pattern we typically use when we're stressed.

Many people find that yoga is a great form of meditation. This ancient form of stretching and exercising trains you to focus on the breath while moving your body into a myriad of poses that help you gain flexibility and strength. You may want to find a class in your area or purchase some of the many books and DVDs that will get you started on a regular routine. Many of my clients swear by yoga as a way to help them relax, reduce back pain, and sleep better.

If you're going through a particularly rough time and you can't change the circumstances, you may need a more powerful form of stress relief, such as hypnosis. I'm not suggesting swinging pocket watches or dancing like a chicken—the sorts of things we see on television or in entertainment shows. The type of hypnosis I'm talking about is like a form of deep meditation that can relieve pain by reaching the depths of your unconscious mind. I recommend a set of CDs called Hypnosis: The Pain Solution. This great product, developed by Dr. Maggie Phillips, guides you through 10 exercises that help you learn to reverse the course of chronic pain.

There are a myriad of ways to cope with stress and to process the difficult emotions in your life. What you must not do is ignore your feelings, muddle through them, or think you're strong enough to just stuff them away. It's a process of taking control of pain, rather than allowing it to control you, that determines if you're an owner or a victim. The category you fall into will have significant impact on your level of pain and the way you perceive it.

Owners vs. Victims

Steve Chandler, author of Reinventing Yourself, taught me that there are two types of people: owners and victims. Owners take full responsibility for their outcomes. They know that they are the sole creator of their actions and reactions. Victims, on the other hand, see themselves as being dealt a bad hand. They take no responsibility, placing blame for their circumstances or pain on life, other people, bad luck, or some circumstance that they cannot control.

As it relates to pain, owners know that their beliefs and emotions can intensify or reduce the pain they experience. Instead of laying around, moaning and groaning, they take action to improve their situation. By responding in a positive manner, owners don't allow pain to control them—they prefer to control their pain. Victims are quite the opposite. They succumb to their pain and complain about it, while failing to do anything to reduce the level of pain they endure or improve their health. They become the victim of their pain and allow it to control them and their life.

These two different mindsets can determine the length of time it takes to recover. Victims allow their beliefs and emotions to keep them stuck in pain. Owners, however, say, "Okay, it happened. Now, it's up to me to heal and get on with this wonderful thing called life." There is no victim mentality or blame—simply a response that chooses not to be stuck in pain.

How do you know if you're an owner or a victim? For starters, pay attention to the things you say and think. Do you usually have a positive outlook? You're probably an owner. Do you love life and take advantage of every day that you've been given? That's an owner, too. On the contrary, if you're pessimistic or believe that life, people, and circumstances are out to get you, you're displaying victim tendencies.

Another important aspect of these two types of people is evidenced when they make mistakes. Everybody makes mistakes, but when a victim does, he blames himself or other people, beating himself up about it incessantly. Owners, though, are those who choose to learn from their mistakes, thus gaining something positive from them, and then moving on.

How does all of this relate to back pain? The way a person

responds to pain is a choice. They can own their pain or be a victim of it. The owner approaches it from the standpoint that it's their own responsibility to control their pain. You might hear an owner say, "I want to be pain free, so I'm going to do my exercises, even if it's uncomfortable." The victim, however, might say, "I should do my exercises, but it hurts too much. This is not fair. Why me?" As you can see, the victim is prolonging recovery by staying stuck in their pain, while the owner is taking responsibility and action to get better.

It's all part of our energy and emotions. These things interact with the mind and body, impacting the way we feel. Negative words, thoughts, and energy leave us feeling drained, fatigued, and stressed—all of these things can create even more pain.

Positive words, thoughts, and energy, however, are healers. Think about the last time you felt pain and someone made you laugh. For a brief moment, whatever made you laugh lessened your pain or made you forget about it altogether. In that particular moment, you didn't allow pain to control you—you chose not to dwell on it. Creating positive energy through your thoughts and emotions can promote healing, reduce pain, and significantly impact its effect on your life.

As Steve explained, it's the difference between "What can I do?" and "Who can I blame?" "What can I do?" signifies that you have power over whatever has happened, while "Who can I blame?" places control, as well as the responsibility to fix it, in someone else's hands.

How you respond to a situation, even pain, is a choice. Whether you are an owner or a victim is a choice—your choice. You can make a commitment to reducing your pain, or you can let pain control you and impact your health, your career, your relationships, and happiness. It's your choice. You also have a choice to stay stuck in pain or to own it and take responsibility for your outcomes and health. Changing your emotions and beliefs from victim to owner is an option that will enable you to claim the power over your pain and take the necessary steps toward healing.

If you want to get rid of back pain, experiment with coping techniques, find the ones that work for you, and implement them in your life. If you want to feel better, it's imperative!

Here are some online resources you may want to explore:
- www.visionday.com
- www.clubfearless.net
- www.sedona.com
- www.familyconstellations.net
- www.hypnosisnetwork.com
- www.emofree.com

CHAPTER 19

BALANCE YOUR NUTRITION

From the bitterness of disease man learns
the sweetness of health.
Catalan Proverb

No matter what kind of back pain you're suffering from—tissue-based, nerve-based, or both—you're going to make your situation better by improving your diet. I'm not going to tell you to give up eating the things you love to eat. But I do want to emphasize just how important your nutrition is to your ability to live without pain.

Just try one or more of the tips below. (The more you do, the better you'll feel.) Try it for just seven days and see if it helps you feel better.

Tip #1:
Drink More Water

Water helps the body in so many ways. I mentioned earlier how the discs in the spine are made up mostly of water. When we drink more, we reinflate those discs after they've been depleted throughout the day.

Water helps eliminate toxins from the body and promotes more efficient kidney function. Flushing toxins out on a regular basis can help prevent trigger points from forming and reduce the severity of those already present in the muscle tissues.

Drinking water helps joints function more smoothly, because it cushions the muscles and provides more support for the body's movement. It fills the stomach, which can deter us from eating too much, and helps to keep our energy levels high.

The "eight glasses a day" rule is a good general guideline, but remember, everyone is different. Everyone has a different weight, metabolism, and activity level, so you need to experiment with what's right for you.

Men typically require more water per day than women. People living in warm climates should drink water more often.

As we get older, our bodies are less able to determine when we need more water, so older people should drink on a regular schedule, even if they're not particularly thirsty.

When you're exercising, drink more, as your body will use more. If you sit at a computer several hours a day, make it a point to get up every hour and get another glass of water. Try drinking a full glass before you start your day in the morning and a full glass with dinner at night. Replace sugary soft drinks with water to reduce calorie intake and to keep caffeine from emptying your body of the water it already has.

As I mentioned before, the best way to judge if you're getting enough water is to check the color of your urine. It may not be a glamorous activity, but it's an easy way to see if your body is hydrated. The middle of the day is the best time. A pale yellow to clear color is best, so if you're seeing a deep yellow, drink more.

Consuming healthy amounts of water may not completely eliminate your pain, but it's likely to help.

It's easy, healthy, and free, so why not try it? It's nothing more than a habit. If you spend a week drinking more water, you will very likely find your body feeling better and craving the higher water intake.

Tip #2:
Take a High-Quality
Multivitamin

The best advice for anyone experiencing back problems is to eat a healthy, well-balanced diet. But for many of us, this is a tall order. We often don't have time to cook homemade meals because we're on the go all the time, and even if we do eat a good amount of fruits and vegetables, unless they are organic or we grow them ourselves, we can never be sure of their nutrient content. And even then, most produce is grown in nutritionally depleted soils, so no matter how healthy you eat, you still are likely to have nutritional deficiencies.

So, to give the body the nutrients it needs to help reduce inflammation and ease back pain, I recommend that all my clients take a high-quality multivitamin—emphasis on high quality. There are a lot of pills out there that aren't going to do you much good. Many companies manufacture products that are highly compressed and glued together into hard tablets that can be very difficult for the body to digest.

You can visualize the process. Imagine if you took a bunch of different vitamins in powder form—pressed them all together, slammed it flat, processed it through a bunch of machines, added binding ingredients to keep it together, sprinkled in preservatives so it would last for months on the shelf, and then spit it out as this hardened, rock-like pill. Would your body get much good out of that?

That's how most multivitamins and supplements are produced. The less processing they go through, the better. The problem is, most people just look at the price and go for the cheapest brand. But in the world of supplements, you often get what you pay for. If you want something that's actually going to help your body stay healthy—and help reduce back pain—invest in a product that's highly digestible.

This probably means you're going to have to take more pills to get a full dose. For example, if you don't smash and press all the nutrients together, they take up more volume, and so a full dose will have to be spread across multiple pills. Keep in mind that in these cases your vitamin dosage isn't necessarily higher, it's just uncompressed, which makes it much easier to digest. The vitamins are much more likely to be absorbed by your body. Remember, it's not how many vitamins you ingest that matters, it's how many your body can actually absorb and use.

Look for a quality multivitamin that exceeds the recommended daily allowance of vitamins and minerals, as the RDA is severely inadequate for optimal heath. Avoid those that come in tablet form and choose instead liquids, soft-gel caplets, or capsules.

Tip #3:
Use a Natural Anti-Inflammatory and Pain Reliever

In Chapter 8, I talked about inflammation and how much it contributes to back pain. Our modern day diet, full of processed and nutritionally void foods, triggers an increase of inflammation in our bodies until we're overloaded with it. Inflammation creates pain in our muscles, nerves, and joints, and it is always a big factor in all kinds of back pain.

What we need are more of the nutrients that cool inflammation down (found in fruits, vegetables, nuts, and fish) and more of our own natural anti-inflammatories—the proteolytic enzymes that stop inflammation and clear out scar tissue. Unfortunately, most of us aren't eating enough anti-inflammatory nutrients, and as we get older, our bodies make fewer anti-inflammatory enzymes.

So, first, as I mentioned, we need to eat a healthy diet and take a quality multivitamin in order to give our bodies the nutrients needed to counteract the inflammation response. Second, we need to replenish the body with more of its own natural anti-inflammatory enzymes. When we do this, two things happen: We cool inflammation and we clear out the stiffening scar tissue that it leaves behind. That means less pain and more fluidity in movement, since scar tissue is what makes us feel stiff in the first place.

As I mentioned in Chapter 11, it's best to find a supplement that combines enzymes and herbs in a formula targeted to reduce inflammation and pain. Look at the "other ingredients" listed below the supplement facts and avoid animal derivatives, preservatives, or artificial things like titanium dioxide. Finally, as with multivitamins, look for capsules or gel tabs.

You'll find the product I recommend, Heal-n-Soothe®, at **www.healnsoothe.com.** The ingredients in this formula have tons of clinical studies behind them, as well as hundreds of years of use, so it's a safer bet than a lot of other wannabes on the market.

Tip #4:
Avoid Inflammatory Foods

In Chapter 8, I also mentioned how many of the foods we're eating today actually promote inflammation. You want to avoid eating these as much as possible or at least limit the amount in your daily diet. These include processed foods, fatty foods, high-sugar items, and refined grains.

Processed foods. Foods filled with preservatives and processed with chemicals introduce foreign elements into the body. The immune system sees these ingredients as a threat and revs up inflammation to "defend" against them. In addition, foods stripped of their natural goodness during processing—like white flour—break down too quickly and spike hormone levels, again encouraging inflammation.

Minimize the amount of refined grains you consume, and eat raw fruits and vegetables whenever possible. Frozen fruits and vegetables are a healthy second option. Fresh and frozen meats are much less likely to promote inflammation than those processed in ready-made meals.

Fatty foods. Remember, not all fats are bad for you. But even too much of a good fat is no good. The fats you want to avoid completely are partially or fully hydrogenated fats, trans fats, and vegetable oils. These fats tip the scales toward inflammation, mainly because they throw off the body's natural balance of fats. Reduce your intake of these items and choose instead meats such as grass-fed (and free range) beef, chicken, and turkey; wild-caught (not farm-raised) fish such as salmon, sardines, herring, and cod; nuts such as almonds, walnuts, and cashews; and beans. These types of foods contribute the healthier omega-3 fats, helping the body fight off inflammation. (An omega-3 supplement is also a good idea.)

High-sugar items. High amounts of sugar cause the body to release regulating hormones, which encourage inflammation. Sugar is everywhere in our food supply, so to help reduce back pain, really watch your intake. Drink soft drinks and sugary fruit juices in small amounts (or not at all), and use water, teas (hot and iced), low-sugar coffees (avoid high-impact cappuccinos), almond or rice milk, and seltzer waters instead.

Eat fewer cakes, cookies, doughnuts, candies, sugary cereals, and pies, and try fruit desserts, frozen yogurt, and sugar-free options instead. Finally, look at your everyday foods. Soups, sauces, ketchup, cereals, applesauce, drink mixes, snack bars, and more all can have extra sugar added. Choose organic and sugar-free options. When you do use sugar, look for raw, unrefined varieties.

Refined grains. Processed or refined grains are found in flour, cereals, breads, baked goods, and snack foods. Usually they're listed as "enriched" flour or anything other than "whole." In essence, refined grains have been broken down for you, so your body doesn't have to do the work. Since the grain then breaks down too quickly in the body and the intestines, it releases hormones that promote inflammation.

Choose foods made with whole grains, such as oatmeal; brown rice; and whole-grain breads, cereals, and crackers. Also, you may want to try limiting your intake of grains overall, particularly wheat, as it has been shown to increase inflammation for many people.

Try substituting an apple for your normal midday cracker snack. You'll have eliminated one serving of grains, pushing your diet into a more balanced state. Replace your wheat-based cereal with oatmeal, which tends to be less inflammatory. Instead of bread for lunch, try a salad with fruit and nuts and a side of yogurt. Just one of these adjustments can go a long way toward alleviating pain.

A Better Diet Takes Stress Off Your Back

Four things. That's what I've outlined here. Four simple things you can do today—this week—that will help ease your back pain. These are easy things and they don't take up much time. Drink more water; take a good multivitamin; use an enzyme supplement; and avoid high-fat, high-sugar, and processed foods. Try it for one to two weeks and I'll bet you'll find yourself feeling a lot better. Plus, since tastes change as you eat different foods, you'll probably start to wonder why you ever wanted all those fatty things in the first place.

Watch a free online video for more nutrition
tips that can relieve your back pain.
www.losethebackpain.com/nutrition

PART III:

PAIN RELIEF
ACTION PLANS

CHAPTER 20

GETTING STARTED: 7-DAY ACTION PLANS

Every patient carries her or his own doctor inside.
Albert Schweitzer

I've designed the remainder of this book to be used as a reference. In the following pages, you'll find clear action plans for eight different back pain conditions. Simply choose the one that applies most directly to you, turn to that page, and get started.

Before you start, however, let me tell you a little about these action plans and how they work.

Remember:
Back Pain Can Have
Several Underlying Causes

As I've said throughout this book, back pain can be caused by a lot of things. Problems in the mind, body, and diet all can contribute.

For long-term relief, we have to figure out and address the right causes—and *all* the causes, if possible. If you've read the entire book up to this point, you probably already have a pretty good idea about what factors are contributing to your back pain.

Even if you're still not sure, the good thing about these action plans is that they're more complete than any other approaches

I've seen out there. Each takes you through a series of steps; so if one step doesn't solve the problem, you still have several more to try.

As you go through each part of the plan, make a mental note of your progress. You may even want to use a specific notebook to record your daily observations. Keeping track of your improvement will help you decide when and if you need to add another step to your treatment.

Recipes for Pain Free Living

I like to tell my clients to think of these action plans as recipes. Each has a set of "ingredients" you're going to choose to either add or remove from your personal routine.

For example, everyone is going to start with the first recommended solution, which addresses the most common cause of the condition. If you suffer from lower back pain, for instance, you're going to start with Muscle Balance Therapy, since muscle imbalances are the most common cause of such pain.

After a certain amount of time, you'll want to record your progress. You may be feeling better, but if you're not 100 percent pain free, then it's time to add ingredient #2.

As you add ingredients, you'll be doing so in a cumulative fashion. In other words, you won't get rid of #1 when you add #2. It's like making chicken soup. You start with chicken broth. When you add the vegetables, you add them to the chicken broth, you don't throw the broth away.

So, as you add steps, or ingredients, to your treatment, stay committed to the steps you're already doing. This helps to address the variety of causes that may be contributing to your back pain.

Judge Your Progress in Percentages

To help you to determine your progress, I suggest you measure it in numbers. For example, let's say you try the first step, which may be Muscle Balance Therapy. After the recommended amount of time, ask yourself: How much of my pain has gone away? If you feel 50 percent better, then most likely you'll want to add step #2 to your routine. If, however, you feel 90 percent better, you may want to stick with the first step for another week and then reexamine your progress.

As a rough rule of thumb, the first step—which is usually Muscle Balance Therapy—will completely solve the problem for about 40 percent of people. For another 40 percent or so, it will make it much better but not get rid of it completely. For the final 20 percent, it may not feel like it's helping at all (even if it is).

So for 60 percent of back pain sufferers, step #2 will be necessary. Often, this is trigger point therapy. These individuals will continue Muscle Balance Therapy and add trigger point therapy to their routines. Again, after the recommended amount of time, they'll want to evaluate their progress.

This time, about 60 percent of this group soon will be pain free. About 30 percent will feel even better, but perhaps still have some discomfort. And 10 percent will see little effect.

These are all approximations to help you see how the action plans work. I haven't actually researched the data to come up with specific statistics. But in my practice, I find that this is pretty close to what actually happens.

The Layered Approach to Solving Back Pain

You will likely experience welcome relief using the first few steps. You'll probably be surprised at how quickly your pain goes away. But if you're one of those who have battled with back pain for a long time, the "layered" approach may be the only way to go.

This is usually because your back pain is caused by a multitude of factors and perhaps has become so "normal" for your body that it will take a longer, more comprehensive approach to break the cycle.

The key is to use the treatments suggested, in the order suggested, at the same time until you can figure out the right combination that works for you. Once you have it figured out, you can stop using the treatments that you suspect aren't as effective, thereby arriving at the simplest possible solution.

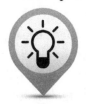 Here's a big tip: Add or subtract treatments one at a time. Add only one treatment at a time. Subtract them one at a time. You want to figure out how each treatment is impacting your pain level. If you add several treatments all at once and the pain goes away, you won't know which one worked the best.

Instead, keep adding one treatment at a time until the entire problem is resolved. Then, slowly remove treatments that seemed to be least effective—again, one at a time. By doing this in a systematic fashion, you can zero in on the precise treatment combination that works best for your specific situation.

Finally, remember what worked for you. To keep back pain away permanently generally takes some light maintenance. I've worked with enough clients to know that when people's lives get busy, they revert back to old habits. For example, if you learned to relax and eat better and your pain went away, don't be surprised if, when you forget to relax and start eating bad foods again, your pain returns.

The same goes for the physical therapies, such as Muscle Balance Therapy. Once you've gotten your muscles rebalanced, it doesn't take much to keep them that way. But if you neglect them—for example, by sitting in a chair 10 hours straight for several days in a row, without standing up, walking around, or stretching—the problem will come back.

If that happens, it's not the end of the world. Just remember which recipe worked best for you and you can fix the problem within a few days.

If you're really in tune with your body, mind, and diet, you often can predict when your bad habits are about to reach a breaking point, as little twinges of back pain will sometimes (but not always) precede you "throwing out" your back.

Again, this "see how close to the edge you can get without falling over" approach isn't what I recommend. But I realize that sometimes old habits sneak back in, so this is a practical approach to managing your back pain and keeping it from getting in the way of your life.

Use the Rest of the Book as Needed

As you review the steps in each of the upcoming action plans, feel free to go back to earlier chapters for more information.

For example, if your action plan specifies you try trigger point therapy, you may want to review Chapter 16. You'll find product recommendations and explanations that will help you get the most out of this step.

Remember to take your time and invest in your own health. Your relief may come quickly, but that isn't the case for everyone. For some people, back pain takes a long time—sometimes years—to develop, so it's logical to assume that in these cases it will take some time to properly correct it.

The good news is that once you've adopted these steps into your daily routine, you will have incorporated an arsenal of tools you can use not only to feel better now, but also to arm yourself for correcting any future back pain episodes, should they appear later in life.

You may even find yourself enjoying the benefits so much that you keep many of the steps in your daily routine, even after your back pain has disappeared. If that's the case, you'll probably help prevent any future back pain episodes.

CHAPTER 21

SUMMARY OF PRIMARY TREATMENT OPTIONS

*"I must do something" always solves more problems
than "Something must be done."*
Author Unknown

We've come to the point where you now can begin implementing solutions to your back pain problems. Following is a summary of five treatment options, each of which you may use in your own recovery. To determine which to use, and when, in your own personalized program, refer to the upcoming chapters.

By now you probably have a pretty good idea about what is causing your back pain. If you have a herniated disc, for example, refer to Chapter 26, which will tell you which of the following options to start with and how long to continue before adding any of the other options. If you have sciatica, refer to Chapter 27; scoliosis, Chapter 28; and so on.

For each pain condition, the order of treatments may vary, so be sure to glance through the chapter that most closely fits your condition before beginning any of the treatments. Also, if you're currently experiencing too much pain to implement any of the therapies below, the chapter on your particular condition will guide you through some short-term pain relief solutions to help you feel better. As soon as you feel ready, begin your personalized treatment program.

Option #1: Muscle Balance Therapy

Muscle Balance Therapy is an approach that works for everyone—regardless of the condition your doctor may have diagnosed—because we all have muscle imbalances. For many people, Muscle Balance Therapy is all that's needed. For others, additional treatments may be necessary. As I mentioned earlier, very rarely is back pain caused by one thing; instead, it's often the result of a combination of causes. Therefore, your treatment plan should include a combination of treatments.

Today's more sedentary lifestyle tends to create muscle imbalances in the torso, hips, and thighs—leading to numerous cases of lower back pain. Some of the muscles are used too much and others too little, while sitting for hours constricts circulation, causing blood to flow too slowly. All this puts pressure on the spine, pulls vertebrae out of alignment, pinches nerves, and also contributes to painful trigger points.

For a review on muscle imbalances, see Chapter 6. To get started on Muscle Balance Therapy, see Chapter 15 or find out how to get your own personalized self-diagnostic and treatment system at **www.losethebackpain.com/getstarted.**

Option #2: Trigger Point Therapy

After one to two weeks of using Muscle Balance Therapy, if you're still experiencing pain, it's time to add trigger point therapy to your routine. Trigger point therapy can help eliminate muscle pain and spasms that Muscle Balance Therapy may not have been able to address. However, don't stop the Muscle Balance Therapy, as it does many things for you that trigger point therapy can't, such as strengthen weak muscles; lengthen short, tight muscles; work to correct imbalances; and, most important, eliminate the dysfunction.

Remember that trigger points can be persistent points of pain, and because of their position in the muscle fibers, they can keep you feeling stiff and sore. Just a few minutes on the trigger point platform I recommended in Chapter 16 can bring you the relief you need for a full recovery. Gravity works for you by applying gentle pressure to the trigger points, thereby loosening them up, relaxing chronically tight muscle fibers, and releasing built-up toxins.

For a review of trigger points and my recommended treatments for them, see Chapter 16. You can find the trigger point solution I recommend at **www.losethebackpain.com/triggerpoints**.

Option #3: Spinal Decompression

After two weeks of combined Muscle Balance Therapy and trigger point therapy, if you still aren't completely pain free, it's time to add spinal decompression therapy to your routine.

I've found in my practice that combining spinal decompression therapy with Muscle Balance Therapy is a very effective way to relieve all kinds of back pain. Often, when Muscle Balance Therapy and trigger point therapy aren't enough to get you to 100 percent, the problem is a disc that's still bulging enough to put pressure on a nerve somewhere in the spine.

Muscle Balance Therapy rebalances the muscles so they no longer pull the spine out of alignment, but that alone may not be enough to allow the discs to "pop" back into place or provide enough of an increase in blood flow to promote healing. In other words, your muscles are probably closer to properly supporting your back, but the vertebrae may need some assistance in getting back to their ideal position, where they'll no longer impact the nerves.

This is where spinal decompression therapy can be extremely effective. Since the human body is upright most of the time, gravity is constantly placing downward pressure on the spine, which is referred to as "compression." Turning the body upside down allows gravity to pull the spine in the opposite direction, opening up the spaces between the vertebrae—which often encourages the discs to return to a healthy position and, if torn, heal themselves. Again, a few minutes a day of this therapy can be enough to help you start experiencing significant relief. And with literally millions of success stories, it's definitely something you'll want to consider.

There are several types of spinal decompression, each a different technique which creates a different effect on the body. Let's take a look at them and their outcomes.

Inversion Therapy

Inversion therapy works on the principle that, by turning your body upside down (or inverting your body), you are able to reverse the effects of gravity on your spine. The weight of your head, neck, and shoulders pulls your spine, opening it just enough that the misaligned discs can be sucked back into their proper place and away from the nerves.

This practice of hanging upside down can be safely done on an inversion table in your own home. Relief is often felt immediately, so it provides both short- and long-term benefit to back pain sufferers.

There are many different inversion tables available in the marketplace. I suggest you look for one that is quality made and manufactured, which provides different degrees of inversion, and one which comes with good reviews and customer support.

The Back Ease is similar to an inversion table in that it uses a spinal decompression technique to reduce pain and create traction to realign the spine. Not a table, it's a device that stabilizes a person and allows them to lean forward, tilting the upper portion of their body downward. The user controls the position of the body to produce the amount of traction that works best for them.

The Back Ease is recommended for most causes and types of

back pain, including lower back pain, sciatica, scoliosis, SI joint dysfunction, stenosis, and degenerative or herniated discs. It also claims to relieve hip pain and pain generated from arthritis, as well as many other diseases and injuries.

Manual Distraction

The second type of spinal decompression is called manual distraction. Manual distraction is performed on a table that allows the therapist to focus specifically on one particular area of the spine. The therapist pulls on the spine, pulling on one joint at a time. Manual distraction is recommended for people with herniated discs, sciatica, and similar problems that produce back pain.

Mechanical Pelvic Traction

One of the most common spinal decompression techniques, mechanical pelvic traction pulls the body, similar to traditional traction that's used in hospitals. The legs are positioned at a 90-degree angle to the upper body, while the body is pulled inter-mittently or continuously. Each treatment lasts approximately 10 to 20 minutes, and with each additional session, the amount of pull is gradually increased.

Immediate relief can be achieved through mechanical pelvic traction, but the longest lasting results are usually obtained with ongoing treatments.

Which of these spinal decompression techniques are best? That is individual, based on a person's unique pain, the cause of the pain, their response to the technique, and other factors like cost and convenience.

An inversion table or alternative spinal decompression device like the Back Ease costs several hundred dollars, but can be used at home and will probably never have to be replaced. Manual dis-traction and pelvic traction each require a visit to a therapist and the accompanying per visit fees. One consideration in determining which technique is best for you is whether you're seeking short-term treatment or want to use spinal decompression as one part of an overall plan to prevent and eliminate back pain for life.

For a review of spinal decompression therapy, see Chapter 17. For the inversion table I use, go to **www.losethebackpain.com/ inversion**. You can also learn more about the Back Ease by going to: **www.losethebackpain.com/backease**.

Option #4: Emotional Troubleshooting

If you've used the combination of Muscle Balance Therapy, trigger point therapy, and spinal decompression therapy for several weeks and you're still experiencing pain, it may be time to evaluate your emotional state of mind.

I've found that, in most cases, if someone is not feeling a lot better by the time they've adopted these three therapies—particularly if the person is doing them diligently on a daily basis—the problem is often a case of severe stress and, in some extreme cases, lingering anger from some emotional trauma (e.g., divorce, abuse, abandonment).

This is when I talk to my client and encourage a serious evaluation of the stresses in his or her life. What I find, more often than not, are job pressures, relationship issues, health concerns (if the person is dealing with a serious disease or troubling diagnosis), significant losses, career confusion, or family troubles.

In some cases, the client has to go a little deeper and ask himself, "Is some past trauma causing my pain?" An old emotional injury can cause a lot of damage, particularly if you haven't thought about it for a while or repressed it in the past.

Evaluate the stresses in your life and see if you can reduce some of them. If you suspect an old trauma may be affecting you, consider an appointment with a licensed therapist. At the very least, carve out some personal time to reflect and record your thoughts, talk to a trusted friend, or purchase some helpful books—anything that might help you get to the core of your pain.

Also, it's important to point out that you don't need to wait to address your mindset, beliefs, and emotions. In fact, I encourage you to begin this process as soon as you begin the other treatments, as your state of mind will have an impact on how well the physical treatments work for you. For example, if you are in a negative state of mind, you actually can prevent proven treatments from working. Don't be one of the people who says, "It didn't work for me," because you (or your mind) wouldn't let it work for you.

For more information on back pain caused by negative stress and emotions, see Chapter 7. For tips on what you can do about "emotional imbalances," see Chapter 18.

Option #5: Dietary Adjustments

If you've gotten to this point and you're still experiencing pain, don't lose hope. Your diet could have a lot to do with it.

First, let me encourage you to continue with the four steps outlined above. Some people with particularly stubborn, chronic back pain just need to hang in there a little longer to see results. Remember, your back pain took a long time to develop and it may just need more time to right itself—especially if you have a very stubborn case. This is particularly true if you have a lot of causes contributing to the pain, such as muscle imbalances, trigger points, bulging discs, and emotional stressors. And don't be surprised if that's the case, as it's actually very common to have numerous causes, some of which require a lot of digging to uncover.

Continue with the previous four steps and, in addition, start adjusting your diet. Though diet usually doesn't cause back pain all by itself, it can certainly make existing back pain worse or create conditions in the body that make it harder to heal. Sometimes, diet is what pushes your pain level "over the edge" to the point where you can really feel it.

You may be eating a lot of things that could be increasing the inflammation in your muscles and nerves. If you're overweight, the extra pounds could be making it more difficult to rebalance your muscles. Your diet also could be increasing the toxins in your system, contributing to trigger points.

For example, even if you're doing trigger point therapy every night, if you're then eating foods that put more toxins back into your body during the day, you'll just be maintaining your current condition, rather than improving it. You may not be drinking enough water, which could be depriving your discs of the shock absorption they need or contributing to toxic buildup in your muscles.

Changing your diet could be the one thing you need to tip the scales in favor of your recovery. Your body needs good, wholesome food to give it the strength and power it needs to heal. And just like with emotional changes, you can implement dietary changes at the very beginning of your treatment program and continue choosing more healthful foods as you work on the physical treatments.

For more information on how your diet is contributing to your pain, see Chapter 8. For tips on how to adjust your diet to reduce pain, see Chapter 19.

Getting Started

I encourage you to get started with your self-treatment plan today. With just a little bit of effort, you can achieve long-lasting back pain relief. In addition to this book, you can find numerous free videos and articles on reducing pain, including condition-specific information, treatment plans, and in-depth reviews of additional pain relief strategies at my website, **www.losethebackpain.com**.

CHAPTER 22

ADDITIONAL TREATMENT OPTIONS

Make your own recovery the first priority in your life.
Robin Norwood

If you've tried various treatments and techniques but still haven't found the pain relief you're seeking, all hope is not lost. There are several other techniques and therapies that are gaining popularity and providing back pain sufferers with relief when others have failed. Let's take a look at some of them and what they can do.

Frequency Specific Microcurrent

In combination with a proper diagnosis, Frequency Specific Microcurrent (FSM) therapy delivers currents to the afflicted area, sending energy that renews cells and reduces pain. FSM works on biophysics principles, actually altering or changing tissue and reducing inflammation and scarring. Some find immediate relief upon the first treatment, and over time, the pain is eliminated altogether.

FSM is usually delivered in a series of treatments performed on a regular basis. After the desired pain relief has been achieved, the patient can be prescribed a home unit where they can continue self-treatment, if necessary.

Of those that have tried FSM therapy, some have received

relief—others have not. One good thing about the treatment is that even if it doesn't help, it doesn't hurt. So there is virtually no danger of risky side effects to FSM therapy.

FSM has been found to be very effective in treating both muscle and nerve pain, particularly pain caused by disc bulges and nerve traction injuries. Other FSM frequencies have been developed for those suffering with lower back pain, joint and shoulder pain, and disc injuries.

You can learn more about Frequency Specific Microcurrent from one of its leading practitioners, Dr. Carolyn McMakin, and see a video demonstration of its use at **www.losethebackpain.com/fsm**.

Prolozone Therapy

Dr. Frank Shallenberger pioneered Prolozone therapy, a technique which injects oxygen into damaged tissues, joints, ligaments, and tendons. This technique is based on the circulation of blood throughout the body, bringing it vitamins, minerals, and oxygen. Low levels of oxygen can create pain. When oxygen is reintroduced into those areas, healing begins.

Prolozone involves three specific techniques. Injected first are homeopathic anti-inflammatory medications, which reduce inflammation and swelling, thus increasing circulation in the area. Then, specific vitamins and minerals are added to promote healing. The last step is injecting ozone into the afflicted area. The average person needs three to five treatments.

Prolozone has seen success in treating musculoskeletal and joint pain, including chronic neck and back pain, degenerated discs, and shoulder pain, as well as other pain not related to the back or neck. Its effects have been permanent for some—because it corrects what causes the pain in the first place, those with chronic pain have a 75% chance of being pain free forever.

Listen to this FREE audio to learn
more about Prolozone:
www.losethebackpain.com/prolozone

Stem Cell Treatment

A third treatment alternative for those suffering with back pain from degenerated, damaged or herniated intervertebral discs uses stem cells to regenerate the discs. This option does more than remove the pain—it also cures the problem that caused it.

An alternative to risky back surgery, stem cell regeneration was developed in the United Kingdom by Dr. Stephen Richardson. A relatively new procedure, it was discovered in 2006. Among the many benefits is the fact that the body cannot reject the stem cells, because they come from the patient, not a donor.

How does it work? The patient's own mesenchymal stem cells (MSC) are combined with a collagen gel that is surgically implanted into the area. It's safer and less invasive than traditional back surgery and has fewer side effects.

This stem cell treatment does what your body would optimally do on its own, if conditions were right. Those conditions include drinking plenty of water, maintaining a healthy diet with the proper amount of vitamins and minerals, and avoiding stress and negativity—all things which I prescribe in this book.

You can learn more about stem cell therapy and Dr. Richardson's research and work by visiting: **www.losethebackpain.com/stemcells.**

Additional Treatment Options

There are many other treatments available, although the ones I've highlighted in this and the previous chapters have proven to be the most effective. If after you've tried all the above recommendations, don't give up or stop there.

Here's a list of some additional treatments, which by themselves may not be enough, but when added to some or all of the ones previously discussed, may be very helpful:

- Acupuncture/Acupressure
- Energy medicine (Reiki, Jin Shin Jyutsu)
- Bodywork (Tui Na, Rolfing, Feldenkrais)
- Nutritional analysis (blood and urine)

In the following chapters, I'll discuss specific back problems and provide short- and long-term pain relief treatments that are effective for each.

CHAPTER 23

LOWER BACK PAIN ACTION PLAN

Although the world is full of suffering,
it is also full overcoming of it.
Helen Keller

People suffering from general lower back pain usually complain of a dull, aching feeling; a tight, "locked up" sensation that limits movement; or sharp pains. Sometimes these sensations are accompanied by radiating pain in the legs and/or feet. All these symptoms can be caused by imbalances within your physical body, mind (e.g., stress), and/or diet. Lower back pain can also be caused by pulled muscles, disc problems, arthritic conditions, or joint dysfunction. It can either be acute or chronic. Acute pain is that which has occurred recently, and chronic pain is one that you've experienced over a longer period of time.

Trauma (injury) and muscle imbalances are the most common causes of lower back pain. While you would know the precise trauma which caused your pain, you probably wouldn't be aware of the muscle imbalance until it resulted in pain. That's because it happens slowly, over a period of time. Muscle imbalances affect your posture, causing "postural dysfunctions," which may include abnormal alignment of the pelvis and abnormal curvature of the spine. This misalignment causes increased wear and tear on the joints, muscles, and ligaments—even the discs.

Traditional treatments offered by physicians for lower back pain include cortisone injections, muscle relaxants, or non-steroidal anti-inflammatory drugs. Chiropractors and physical therapists may offer spinal mobilization, hot packs, ultrasound, electrical stimulation, and therapeutic exercises. In some instances, surgery is suggested, but I believe it should always be your last option.

Lower back pain caused by muscles imbalances cannot be treated effectively through most of the above treatments. In order to reduce or eliminate the pain, you first have to correct what caused it. The most effective treatment is to correct the muscle imbalance and restore postural balance. This treatment works in relieving lower back pain and in preventing future incidences of it.

The following action plan covers two areas: 1) short-term, temporary pain relief and 2) long-term solutions. I always encourage people to work toward the goal of total pain relief—in other words, no more back pain, period. But if you're too uncomfortable to get through the steps needed for a long-lasting solution, you may want to start with the temporary pain relief options (listed below).

For each category of pain relief (temporary versus long term), I've arranged the solutions in order, with the step likely to help you the most listed first. Start with the solution at the top of the list, and then work your way down only if the pain improves but doesn't completely disappear.

Temporary Pain Relief - Action Plan
(see Chapter 11 for details)

1. Far infrared heat therapy
2. Pain relief cream
3. Natural anti-inflammatory (e.g., proteolytic enzyme supplements)

Long-Term Relief - Action Plan
(see Chapter 21 for details)

1. Muscle Balance Therapy

2. Trigger point therapy

3. Spinal decompression therapy

4. Emotional troubleshooting

5. Dietary adjustments

Find this plan summarized in an easy-to-follow format online at:
www.losethebackpain.com/lowerbackplan

CHAPTER 24

UPPER BACK PAIN ACTION PLAN

A new position of responsibility will usually show a man to be a far stronger creature than was supposed.
William James

If you're suffering from general upper back pain, you're probably having a hard time doing daily activities like driving a car, working at the computer, or even brushing your teeth. You may be experiencing headaches or radiating pain into the arms and/or the shoulder blades. You may have had muscles "lock up," making it nearly impossible to move your head or arms. All these symptoms can be caused by problems with your body (usually muscle trauma or imbalances), mind (e.g., stress), and/or diet—and most likely, they've been building up for quite some time.

This region of our back is quite complex, due to the fact that it contains many joints. When working properly, you can perform everyday tasks with ease—but when pain strikes in the upper back, even the simplest activities can be difficult.

The three most common reasons for upper back pain are trauma, trigger points, and muscle imbalances. With trauma, it's easy to determine what caused the pain; however, in the case of trigger points or muscle imbalances, a person may not be able to pinpoint any one thing that triggered it. That's because postural dysfunctions are often the culprit. These postural dysfunctions cause abnormal alignment of the head and shoulders and abnormal positioning of the joints that lead to increased wear and tear on the joints, muscles, and ligaments—even discs. The key to treating upper back pain due to postural dysfunctions is to correct the dysfunction.

It's important to understand that while upper back pain caused by postural dysfunctions or muscle imbalances can introduce itself suddenly, it probably took a long time to develop before any pain was perceived. This is also true of trigger points, which can occur after toxins build up in tissues, muscles, tendons, or ligaments for a period of time.

Common treatments employed by medical professionals include cortisone injections, prescriptions for muscle relaxants or non-steroidal anti-inflammatory drugs, and bed rest. Chiropractic care and physical therapy can offer spinal mobilizations, hot packs, ultrasound, electrical stimulation, cervical traction, and therapeutic exercises. Most of these treatments, though, fail to address the cause of the pain, so while a person may get temporary relief, the condition often lurks in the background, waiting to rear its ugly head one more time. The one thing that effectively provides both pain relief and prevention is correcting the postural imbalance which caused the pain in the first place.

The following action plan covers two areas: 1) short-term, temporary pain relief and 2) long-term solutions. I always encourage people to work toward the goal of total pain relief—in other words, no more back pain, period. But if you're too uncomfortable to get through the steps needed for the long-lasting solution, you may want to start with the temporary pain relief options (listed below).

For each category of pain relief (temporary versus long term), I've arranged the solutions in order, with the step likely to help you the most listed first. Start with the solution at the top of the list, and then work your way down only if the pain improves but doesn't completely disappear.

Temporary Pain Relief - Action Plan
(see Chapter 11 for details)

1. Far infrared heat therapy
2. Pain relief cream
3. Natural anti-inflammatory (e.g., proteolytic enzyme supplements)

Long-Term Relief - Action Plan
(see Chapter 21 for details)

1. Muscle Balance Therapy
2. Trigger point therapy
3. Spinal decompression therapy
4. Emotional troubleshooting
5. Dietary adjustments

Find this plan summarized in an easy-to-follow format online at:
www.losethebackpain.com/upperbackplan

CHAPTER 25

NECK PAIN
ACTION PLAN

Pain is weakness leaving the body.
Tom Sobal

Nearly everyone experiences it at some point in their life. Neck pain can result from accidents or injuries, muscle strain or imbalances, and even simple activities which are repeated over time, like sitting, reading, and working at the computer. Our bodies are in a sitting position often throughout the day. We eat, drive, read, watch TV and even work while sitting. This simple act of sitting can cause the head to move forward, which in turn stretches the muscles across the upper back and shoulders. A stretched muscle is a weak muscle, so when the muscles in our upper back are weakened, so, too, are the neck muscles. The symptoms of this include a neck pain, a "kink" in the neck, pain which radiates into the shoulders or head, and sometimes weakness, numbness, or tingling in the neck, shoulders, or arms.

Neck and upper back pain that's derived from muscle imbalances or trauma require more than attention just to the area of the neck or upper back that's affected—to be truly effective, treatment must focus on the entire spine.

You may be able to identify that you have a pulled muscle or whiplash, which is a common injury due to sudden force, such as a car accident. But knowing that doesn't tell you why you're having pain or which muscles might be imbalanced due to over-use or injury. The only way to compensate for muscle weakness or imbalance is to determine which muscles need strengthened. Then you can begin to address the imbalance, as well as the cause of your neck pain, such as activities or posture. It's not enough to relieve the pain—your goal is to prevent it from recurring, too.

Anti-inflammatory medications can also relieve the pain and are often prescribed by physicians and therapists for that purpose. Don't rely on minimizing the pain through pain relievers to fix the problem. I prefer natural anti-inflammatories, like proteolytic enzyme supplements, rather than medications, regardless if they are prescription or over-the-counter.

Unless you're suffering from a specific injury, most neck and upper back pain can be attributed to poor posture or muscle imbalances; therefore, anti-inflammatory medications are a temporary fix. If you don't correct the cause of the problem, it's almost certain that it will return.

There are corrective exercises for any muscle imbalance, as well as ways to strengthen any set of muscles that has weakened over time. It's very important, though, to identify the muscles that are weak, as well as those which are strong. You don't want to further strengthen a muscle if it's too strong. That could result in making a weak muscle even weaker, countering the result you want to achieve. Therefore, it's imperative that you identify your particular muscle imbalances so you can target your corrective regimen directly on the muscle groups which need it.

Once you've identified the muscles causing your neck pain, begin to identify activities which contribute to your problem. These might include such regular activities as leaning forward to read or eat, raising one shoulder to support a phone between your ear and shoulder, or even sleeping in one position all of the time. Eliminate stress, which frequently introduces itself as neck pain because stress causes neck muscles to tighten and clench.

Correct your posture. Drink plenty of water to help those muscles relax and release built-up toxins. Trigger point therapy can also help loosen knotted muscles, bringing relief to the underlying area.

Neck and upper back pain stemming from trauma or injury might require more than Muscle Balance Therapy or trigger point therapy. While it's always a good idea to use Muscle Balance Therapy in any back or neck pain therapy, certain injuries or imbalances may benefit from cervical spinal decompression or inversion therapy, which we discussed in greater detail in Chapters 17 and 21.

The following action plan covers two areas: 1) short-term, temporary pain relief and 2) long-term solutions. I always encourage people to work toward the goal of total pain relief—in other words, no more back or neck pain, period. But if you're too uncomfortable to get through the steps needed for the long-lasting solution, you may want to start with the temporary pain relief options (listed below).

For each category of pain relief (temporary versus long term), I've arranged the solutions in order, with the step likely to help you the most listed first. Start with the solution at the top of the list, and then work your way down only if the pain improves but doesn't completely disappear.

Temporary Pain Relief - Action Plan
(see Chapter 11 for details)

1. Far infrared heat therapy

2. Pain relief cream

3. Natural anti-inflammatory (e.g., proteolytic enzyme supplements)

Long-Term Relief - Action Plan
(see Chapter 21 for details)

1. Muscle Balance Therapy
2. Trigger point therapy
3. Spinal decompression therapy
4. Emotional troubleshooting
5. Dietary adjustments

Find this plan summarized in an easy-to-follow format online at:
www.losethebackpain.com/neckplan

CHAPTER 26

HERNIATED DISC ACTION PLAN

Fractures well cured make us more strong.
Ralph Waldo Emerson

A herniated disc occurs when the outer part of the donut-shaped disc between the vertebrae weakens and the inner part (a gel-like substance) protrudes outward, something like when a balloon is squeezed from one side. Typically, people don't feel any pain until and unless this protrusion touches a nerve. Many people live out their lives with one or more herniated discs and never know it.

If the protrusion does touch or compress a nerve, it usually causes pain in the lower back, radiating down the back of one or both legs and sometimes causing sharp, needling pain in the bottoms of the feet. If the herniated disc is higher up the spine, radiating pain can occur in the arms.

The primary cause of a herniated disc is the excessive compression and torsion that is placed on the spine, which is the result of numerous muscle imbalances throughout the body. In addition, two often overlooked yet major factors are dietary imbalances and negative stress and/or emotions. Herniated disc disease also is referred to as bulging disc, ruptured disc, slipped disc, prolapsed disc, or degenerative disc disease.

Because a herniated disc is a complicated condition, it may

require several types of treatment approaches. For example, while inversion therapy can provide some relief, better results are often found when inversion therapy is combined with Muscle Balance Therapy.

Controlling stress and inflammation is highly suggested in any herniated disc treatment. Strongly consider changing your diet, including healthier foods and drinking plenty of clean water, proteolytic enzyme therapy and daily self-administered trigger point therapy have also provided relief for many.

Far infrared heat is another treatment that deeply penetrates the area, bringing relief, as well as improved blood flow for faster healing.

This condition specifically responds well to spinal decompression, which reduces the pressure on the surrounding nerves, while increasing range of motion and improving circulation to the afflicted area.

The following action plan covers two areas: 1) short-term, temporary pain relief and 2) long-term solutions. I always encourage people to work toward the goal of total pain relief—in other words, no more back pain, period. But if you're too uncomfortable to get through the steps needed for the long-lasting solution, you may want to start with the temporary pain relief options (listed below).

For each category of pain relief (temporary versus long term), I've arranged the solutions in order, with the step likely to help you the most listed first. Start with the solution at the top of the list, and then work your way down only if the pain improves but doesn't completely disappear.

NOTE: In the long-term list of treatment options, spinal decompression therapy appears first. With a herniated disc, getting pressure off the spine is critical to recovery, and turning the body upside down is the best way to do that. Reverse gravity opens the spaces between the vertebrae, giving them room to heal and encouraging them to slide back into place. If you have this condition, invest in a quality inversion table immediately (see **www.losethebackpain.com/inversion** for my recommendation), and begin using it as soon as you can.

Temporary Pain Relief - Action Plan
(see Chapter 11 for details)

1. Far infrared heat therapy
2. Pain relief cream
3. Natural anti-inflammatory (e.g., proteolytic enzyme supplements)

Long-Term Relief - Action Plan
(see Chapter 21 for details)

1. Spinal decompression therapy
2. Muscle Balance Therapy
3. Trigger point therapy
4. Emotional troubleshooting
5. Dietary adjustments

Find this plan summarized in an easy-to-follow format online at: **www.losethebackpain.com/herniateddiscplan**

CHAPTER 27

SCIATICA ACTION PLAN

The most authentic thing about us is our capacity to create, to overcome, to endure, to transform, to love and to be greater than our suffering.
Ben Okri

The term "sciatica" typically refers to a sharp or steady pain that radiates up and down the back of the leg (i.e., through the hamstring), or "sciatic nerve." Pain also can occur in the lower back, buttocks, and feet. This pain has also been described as a burning, tingling, or traveling sensation, either on one side of the body or both sides at the same time. Sometimes, lower back pain is experienced, as well. Most back pain sufferers and even many medical doctors incorrectly consider sciatica a medical condition. In reality, sciatica isn't a condition itself, but rather a symptom of another underlying condition—like a herniated disc, piriformis syndrome, spinal stenosis, or another back problem. Therefore, it is important to find out just what is causing the condition before you can effectively treat it.

Most of the underlying causes of sciatica mentioned above are caused by muscle imbalances that have been getting worse over time. Other problems with your body, mind (e.g., stress), and/or diet all can contribute by making what would otherwise be a low level of pain much worse.

Traditional treatments for sciatica include cortisone injections, non-steroidal anti-inflammatory medication, electrical stimulation, ultrasound and applying hot packs. However, these treatments address only the symptoms, not the underlying cause such as muscle imbalances.

While there are short-term treatments that provide relief, it's important to understand that a long-term sciatica treatment program may require two or more different types of treatment, including far infrared heat, Muscle Balance Therapy, trigger point therapy, spinal decompression therapy (to improve blood flow and reduce pressure on the nerves), and changes to your diet.

The following action plan covers two areas: 1) short- term, temporary pain relief and 2) long-term solutions. I always encourage people to work toward the goal of total pain relief—in other words, no more back or sciatic pain, period. But if you're too uncomfortable to get through the steps needed for the long-lasting solution, you may want to start with the temporary pain relief options (listed below).

For each category of pain relief (temporary versus long term), I've arranged the solutions in order, with the step likely to help you the most listed first. Start with the solution at the top of the list, and then work your way down only if the pain improves, but doesn't completely disappear.

Temporary Pain Relief - Action Plan
(see Chapter 11 for details)

1. Far infrared heat therapy

2. Pain relief cream

3. Natural anti-inflammatory (e.g., proteolytic enzyme supplements)

Long-Term Relief - Action Plan
(see Chapter 21 for details)

1. Muscle Balance Therapy
2. Trigger point therapy
3. Spinal decompression therapy
4. Emotional troubleshooting
5. Dietary adjustments

Find this plan summarized in an easy-to-follow format online at:
www.losethebackpain.com/sciaticaplan

CHAPTER 28

SCOLIOSIS
ACTION PLAN

Do not yield to misfortunes, but meet them on
the contrary with fortitude.
Virgil

Scoliosis describes a curvature of the spine—instead of going straight up and down, it curves laterally to one side or the other between the neck and the tailbone. Signs of scoliosis include a shoulder blade that juts out, uneven shoulders or hips, a noticeable leaning to one side, or a rolling walking gait. Symptoms can include tiredness, joint strain, and back pain.

This problem can be caused by many things, including abnormal muscles or nerves, spina bifida, cerebral palsy, bone abnormalities present at birth, injury, illness, previous surgery, or osteoporosis. However, mild scoliosis is most commonly caused by muscle imbalances. As we discussed earlier in this book, muscle imbalances pull the spine out of alignment and can create a lateral curvature.

Often diagnosed during childhood or the early teen years, it's reported that approximately 2 to 3 percent of American 16-year-olds have scoliosis. A very small percentage of those (1/10th of 1 percent) have a curvature extreme enough to warrant surgery. Girls are more likely to be afflicted with scoliosis than boys, though no one quite knows the reason why.

A brace is a common treatment for those with a spinal curve

between 25 and 40 degrees and who still have two or more years of growth. The purpose of the brace is to stop the curvature from increasing. Sometimes, the brace does provide temporary correction; however, when it is removed, the curve often returns to its original condition.

If surgery is warranted, it also serves as a measure to stop further curvature, but it does not correct any curvature that has already occurred. Even with surgery, it's likely that perfect alignment of the spine will not occur. A brace may still be needed after surgery, as well as other treatment regimens. The treatment plan that follows is designed to address scoliosis caused by imbalanced muscles. As a child, I was diagnosed with a mild case of scoliosis. My doctor wasn't sure why I had it, but in evaluating the curvature of my back, he noticed it deviated from what was considered typical.

Many years later, as I learned more about the role of muscle balance in back pain, I unintentionally "cured" my scoliosis by rebalancing the muscles in my back and upper body. I discovered that my particular case of scoliosis was caused by lifestyle factors, not the major medical conditions often associated with the condition.

If you've seen a medical doctor and have determined your scoliosis is not caused by a major medical issue, then the following action plan can help you, as it addresses scoliosis caused by lifestyle factors.

This action plan covers two areas: 1) short-term, temporary pain relief and 2) long-term solutions. I always encourage people to work toward the goal of total pain relief—in other words, no more back pain, period. But if you're too uncomfortable to get through the steps needed for the long-lasting solution, you may want to start with the temporary pain relief options (listed below).

For each category of pain relief (temporary versus long term), I've arranged the solutions in order, with the step likely to help you the most listed first. Start with the solution at the top of the list, and then work your way down only if the pain improves but doesn't completely disappear.

Temporary Pain Relief - Action Plan
(see Chapter 11 for details)

1. Far infrared heat therapy

2. Pain relief cream

3. Natural anti-inflammatory (e.g., proteolytic enzyme supplements)

Long-Term Relief - Action Plan
(see Chapter 21 for details)

1. Muscle Balance Therapy

2. Trigger point therapy

3. Spinal decompression therapy

4. Emotional troubleshooting

5. Dietary adjustments

Find this plan summarized in an easy-to-follow format online at:
www.losethebackpain.com/scoliosisplan

CHAPTER 29

SPINAL STENOSIS
ACTION PLAN

We acquire the strength we have overcome.
Ralph Waldo Emerson

Spinal stenosis is a condition in which the spinal canal narrows, compressing or "squeezing" the spinal cord and nerves inside. ("Stenosis" means "narrowing" in Greek.) Most commonly, the narrowing occurs in the lower back, which is called "lumbar spinal stenosis." (When it occurs in the neck, it's called "cervical spinal stenosis.")

Pain exists, however, only if and when the narrowing affects the nerves. If a nerve is touched or squeezed by the spinal canal, pain can occur in the back, legs, neck, arms, and hands, all depending on the location of the narrowing. Numbness or tingling in the legs and feet are also possible, as well as cramps in the legs. The pain usually lessens if you lean forward.

These symptoms can occur intermittently, depending on if and when the nerves are affected. Other problems with the body (muscle imbalances), mind (e.g., stress), and/or diet all can make this condition worse.

Considered an aging disease, spinal stenosis usually occurs in people over 40 years old. While age is a factor, there are two other factors that often are overlooked: the calcification of the spinal canal, which is primarily caused by a nutrient imbalance; and a build-up of fibrin (scar tissue) brought on by a reduction in proteolytic enzymes in the body as we age. The good news is that both of these things can be addressed fairly easily.

For some, spinal stenosis is congenital, caused by imperfections in the development of the spine. Other causes include a herniated disc, osteoporosis, or a tumor.

Traditional treatments for spinal stenosis usually include restriction of movement—in other words, bed rest. Some professionals may recommend corticosteroid injections to minimize swelling, as well as non-steroidal anti-inflammatory drugs and/or acetaminophen. Therapeutic exercises, hot packs, and electrical stimulation may also provide some relief. For those who do not respond favorably to these treatments, surgery may be recommended.

There are additional treatments, though, which have provided pain relief for many people afflicted with spinal stenosis. Everyone with spinal stenosis has trigger points, so daily trigger point therapy is beneficial. To receive maximum benefit, follow trigger point therapy immediately with muscle balance therapy, which helps to return balance and proper function of the joints and muscles.

The deep penetration of far infrared heat therapy has also given some immense relief and improved range of motion, as well as the benefits from improved blood flow to the afflicted area. Ice and/or heat can also help with any inflammation, pain, or stiffness that often accompanies spinal stenosis. Again, some people may gain relief from just one of these treatments, while others may need to implement several of them into their treatment plan.

The following action plan covers two areas: 1) short-term, temporary pain relief and 2) long-term solutions. I always encourage people to work toward the goal of total pain relief—in other words, no more back pain, period. But if you're too uncomfortable to get through the steps needed for the long-lasting solution, you may want to start with the temporary pain relief options (listed below).

For each category of pain relief (temporary versus long term), I've arranged the solutions in order, with the step likely to help you the most listed first.

Start with the solution at the top of the list, and then work your way down only if the pain improves but doesn't completely disappear.

Temporary Pain Relief - Action Plan
(see Chapter 11 for details)

1. Far infrared heat therapy

2. Pain relief cream

3. Natural anti-inflammatory (e.g. proteolytic enzyme supplements)

Long-Term Relief - Action Plan
(see Chapter 21 for details)

1. Nutrient supplementation (see note below)

2. Muscle Balance Therapy

3. Trigger point therapy

4. Spinal decompression therapy

5. Emotional troubleshooting

6. Dietary adjustments

Find this plan summarized in an easy-to-follow format online at:
www.losethebackpain.com/stenosisplan

Nutrient Supplementation

For this condition, it's imperative you begin nutrient supplementation immediately. First, if you haven't already, start with an enzyme supplement. As the body ages, it produces fewer of its own natural fibrin fighters—called proteolytic enzymes. Without these critical enzymes to "eat up" and help wash away scar tissue, it builds up around the discs, contributing to the narrowing of the spine. Supplementing your diet with additional enzymes will help your body to clear away the scar tissue and give your spine back the flexibility it needs to function pain free. These enzymes also act as the body's natural anti-inflammatories, which help prevent fibrin from forming in the first place. For the supplement I recommend, go to **www.healnsoothe.com**.

Second, you need to address the nutrient imbalance that often contributes to the calcification of the spinal canal—namely, an imbalance in calcium, magnesium, and vitamin D. A hair tissue mineral analysis can help you identify any mineral imbalances you have as well as indicate your overall nutritional profile and exposure to toxic elements.

CHAPTER 30

SACROILIAC JOINT DYSFUNCTION ACTION PLAN

The gem cannot be polished without friction,
nor man perfected without trials.
Dutch Proverb

The sacroiliac (SI) joint connects the base of the spine to the pelvis. In other words, it joins the sacrum (the triangular bone at the bottom of the spine) with the pelvis at two connection points. (You can see these from the outside as two "dimples" on each side of the lower back, at the belt line.) It's small, but very strong, remains fairly still, and acts as a shock-absorbing structure.

Because it is a weight-bearing joint, the SI joint can become irritated and inflamed. Oftentimes, muscle imbalances can pull it completely out of alignment. Other causes of SI joint dysfunction can include multiple pregnancies (that have stressed the joint) or one leg that is shorter than the other, as well as imbalances in the mind (e.g., too much negative stress) and the diet (e.g., too much calcium, not enough magnesium). Pain usually occurs in the lower back, with pain radiating to the buttocks and legs. The symptoms may mimic the symptoms of a herniated disc or sciatic pain (pain along the sciatic nerve that radiates down the leg).

Usually, sacroiliac joint dysfunction is the result of an imbalance in the position of the pelvis as it relates to the curvature at the base of the spine. Should the pelvis tip or tilt, the connection points of the joints will be off, causing uneven wear and tear. If left untreated, arthritis can occur in the joint.

Sacroiliac Joint Dysfunction does not occur overnight. It is the result of years of muscle and posture imbalances which ultimately prevent the muscles, bones and SI joint from working together, like they're supposed to do.

Proper treatment requires correcting the muscle imbalances which caused the condition in the first place. Again, it's important to understand that because this condition did not occur suddenly, it will take time to reverse the muscle imbalances—therefore, it can be beneficial to include both the short- and long-term treatments suggested below.

The following action plan covers two areas: 1) short-term, temporary pain relief and 2) long-term solutions. I always encourage people to work toward the goal of total pain relief—in other words, no more back pain, period. But if you're too uncomfortable to get through the steps needed for the long-lasting solution, you may want to start with the temporary pain relief options (listed below).

For each category of pain relief (temporary versus long term), I've arranged the solutions in order, with the step likely to help you the most listed first. Start with the solution at the top of the list, and then work your way down only if the pain improves but doesn't completely disappear.

 If you have SI joint dysfunction, this free video demonstrates rebalancing techniques specific to your condition. Watch it at:
www.losethebackpain.com/sijoint

Temporary Pain Relief - Action Plan
(see Chapter 11 for details)

1. Far infrared heat therapy

2. Pain relief cream

3. Natural anti-inflammatory (e.g., proteolytic enzyme supplements)

Long-Term Relief - Action Plan
(see Chapter 21 for details)

1. Muscle Balance Therapy

2. Trigger point therapy

3. Spinal decompression therapy

4. Emotional troubleshooting

5. Dietary adjustments

Find this plan summarized in an easy-to-follow format online at:
www.losethebackpain.com/sijointplan

CHAPTER 31

OTHER CONDITIONS

*You can't cross the sea merely by standing
and staring at the water.*
Rabindranath Tagore

If you don't have any of the other conditions discussed in this section (Chapters 23-30), you'll most likely find relief by going through the steps in the following action plan. Most back pain situations that don't fall into the other categories still are the result of problems in the mind, body, and/or diet—all of which are addressed here. You will be performing your own self-assessment as you go through the steps, which will help you determine exactly what you need to do to feel better, and it also may help point you to one of the other chapters as you learn more about your own condition.

The following action plan covers two areas: 1) short-term, temporary pain relief and 2) long-term solutions. I always encourage people to work toward the goal of total pain relief—in other words, no more back pain, period. But if you're too uncomfortable to get through the steps needed for the long-lasting solution, you may want to start with the temporary pain relief options (listed below).

For each category of pain relief (temporary versus long term), I've arranged the solutions in order, with the step likely to help you the most listed first. Start with the solution at the top of the list, and then work your way down only if the pain improves but doesn't completely disappear.

Temporary Pain Relief - Action Plan
(see Chapter 11 for details)

1. Far infrared heat therapy

2. Pain relief cream

3. Natural anti-inflammatory (e.g., proteolytic enzyme supplements)

Long-Term Relief - Action Plan
(see Chapter 21 for details)

1. Muscle Balance Therapy

2. Trigger point therapy

3. Spinal decompression therapy

4. Emotional troubleshooting

5. Dietary adjustments

Find this plan summarized in an easy-to-follow format online at:
www.losethebackpain.com/generalplan

CHAPTER 32

YOUR PAIN FREE LIFE

You have to accept whatever comes and the only important thing is that you meet it with courage and with the best that you have to give.
Eleanor Roosevelt

You now have all the tools you need to begin your journey to a pain free life.

I won't wish you luck, as you only need consistent implementation of the treatments to feel better, but I will wish you commitment to your own health and happiness. If you need more information or additional help, please don't hesitate to contact my team at **www.losethebackpain.com**.

Here's to a pain free life!

CHAPTER 33

RECOMMENDED BOOKS AND RESOURCES

Here is a list of recommend resources to alleviate the short- and long-term causes of back pain:

Short-Term Pain Relief Treatments

- **Natural pain relief supplements**
  www.healnsoothe.com

- **Pain relief creams**
  www.rubonrelief.com

- **Far infrared heat therapy**
  www.losethebackpain.com/heat

Long-Term Pain Relief Treatments

- **Muscle Balance Therapy**
  www.losethebackpain.com/muscleimbalances

- **Trigger point therapy**
  www.losethebackpain.com/triggerpoints

- **Inversion therapy**
  www.losethebackpain.com/inversion

For additional updates to this resource list, sign up for my free e-mail newsletter at **www.losethebackpain.com**.

Recommended Reading

The Trigger Point Therapy Workbook - Clair Davies

Healing Back Pain - Dr. John Sarno

The Anti-Inflammation Diet and Recipe Book - Dr. Jessica Black

The Calcium Lie - Dr. Robert Thompson

The Calcium Lie II - Dr. Robert Thompson

Power Sleep - Dr. James Maas

Shift Your Mind - Steve Chandler

The Story of You - Steve Chandler

Pain Relief Products

Lose the Back Pain® System
www.losethebackpain.com/getstarted

Rub on Relief®
www.rubonrelief.com

Inversion Table
www.losethebackpain.com/inversion

Heal-n-Soothe®
www.healnsoothe.com

Lose the Neck Pain™ System
www.losetheneckpain.com

Lose the Back Pain® System

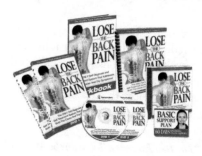

Get rid of your back pain for good. Join over 72,471 people who've erased back pain and sciatica from their lives.

"Long story short.... I've been pain free for the last 8 weeks. And I mean PAIN FREE for the first time in over 15 years!" - Mark A.

Heal-n-Soothe®

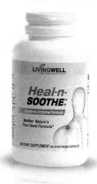

Heal-n-Soothe® is a combination of the most powerful natural anti-inflammatory and pain relieving ingredients known to man... and have been scientifically proven to work. And unlike NSAIDs, there are no dangerous side effects...

Rub On Relief

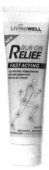

Rub it on and your muscle pain is gone! Just ask people who've tried it...

"Sore, stiff back pain - GONE in Minutes!"
Joey Avantaggio, Bremen, MA

"Immediate relief from my hip pain and muscle spasms"
Margaret Franz, CO

www.losethebackpain.com/products

The Healthy Back Institute's
Premium Inversion Table

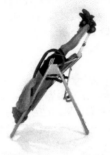

Inversion therapy has been proven to reduce or eliminate various types of back pain. In fact, a recent study found that over 70% of patients who used inversion therapy were able to cancel their back surgery.

"The Best Inversion Table on the Market"

Back Ease

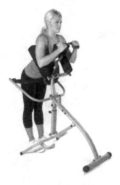

The Back Ease is an excellent way to decompress the spine and is a great alternative to using an inversion table. Order yours today and see just how effective this simple device can be.

Far Infrared Heating Pad

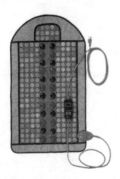

Get the ultimate in deep, penetrating heat with this 21st century heating pad. Pain just melts away because deep, penetrating heat delivers more oxygen-rich blood to painful areas and speeds up your body's natural healing process. It works wonders.

www.losethebackpain.com/products

Love This Book?

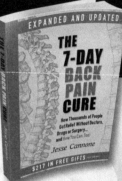

Help others get relief by
sharing your success story...

Our goal is to give away 1 MILLION copies
of this book and we feel that once we
hit that goal, we will have made a huge
impact on how back pain is treated.

**Please take a minute to tell others how
The 7-Day Back Pain Cure helped you.**

Send us your story online:
www.losethebackpain.com/mystory

Or you can fax or mail your story to us:

**Healthy Back Institute
141 E. Mercer St, Suite E
Dripping Springs, TX 78620**

Fax: 1-866-843-4319

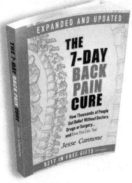

Jesse Cannone

Recognized as one of the leading back pain relief experts in the United States, Jesse Cannone has been helping people eliminate their pain and regain control of their lives for more than a decade. He is an amazing example of how far passion, drive and determination can take you.

Most people would have been content with being a highly successful personal trainer and post-rehabilitation specialist with a thriving fitness business in the Greater Washington, D.C., area. But when Jesse saw that so many of the clients who came to him were suffering with lower back pain and sciatica, he made a decision that would not only change his life but the lives of millions of others - from Atlanta, Georgia, all the way to Queensland, Australia.

That decision was to focus his attention on helping the millions of people who struggle with back pain, neck pain and sciatica. Then, with the help of massage therapist Steve Hefferon and a hand-picked board of medical advisors, he created the world's first self-assessment and self-treatment program for back pain and sciatica sufferers. The system, which is called Lose The Back Pain®, has proven extremely effective and over 65,000 copies have already been sold in over 100 countries.

Having personally worked with hundreds of clients, Jesse has developed a no-nonsense approach to fitness and wellness that has helped people all over the world weed through all the weight loss and fitness hype to discover what really works.

As a result, Jesse has been able to help millions of people reach their weight loss and fitness goals through his articles, books, audio programs, videos, and seminars. In addition to being a certified fitness trainer, bestselling author, and national fitness presenter, he also holds many other certifications, such as Post-Rehabilitation Specialist, Specialist in Performance Nutrition, Advanced Level Fitness Trainer and Master Fitness Trainer. He is also a highly skilled marketing consultant and has helped thousands of other fitness trainers and small businesses to launch, build and grow successful businesses.

His articles and advice now appear on thousands of web sites each month. Jesse has been featured in dozens of magazines and newspapers, including Entrepreneur, Woman's World, Men's Fitness, Balance, Natural Bodybuilding, and The Washington Examiner, and has appeared as a guest on a variety of radio and television programs across the country.

Jesse believes that one of the keys to his success has been his philosophy of always delivering more than he promises and giving every client a WOW experience that they can't wait to tell their friends about.

Jesse and his wife have eight children.

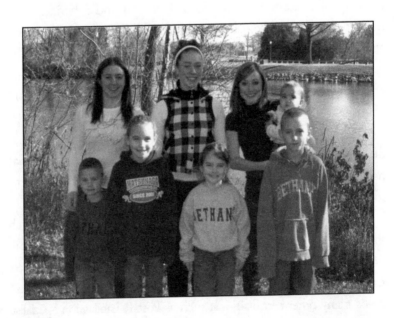